To
Pamela and Amy

Ethics
and the
New Medicine

Ethics
and the
New Medicine

Harmon L. Smith

 abingdon press - nashville and new york

ETHICS AND THE NEW MEDICINE

Copyright © 1970 by Abingdon Press

All rights in this book are reserved.
No part of the book may be reproduced in any
manner whatsoever without written permission of
the publishers except brief quotations embodied in
critical articles or reviews. For information address
Abingdon Press, Nashville, Tennessee

ISBN 0-687-12013-6

Library of Congress Catalog Card Number: 76-124756

SET UP, PRINTED, AND BOUND BY
THE PARTHENON PRESS, AT NASHVILLE,
TENNESSEE, UNITED STATES OF AMERICA

Contents

Preface

My earliest recollection of doctors and medicine was almost my last one. While I was visiting my grandparents in Ellisville, a small town in southern Mississippi, I suffered an onset of excruciating abdominal pain. My grandfather, who spent his professional lifetime in general practice, initially diagnosed the problem as an upset stomach. When the pain persisted the following day, he thought I had perhaps contracted a severe case of food poisoning and prescribed an emetic: in this case, a solid dose of calomel! My real problem, it turned out, was acute appendicitis. But the calomel did its work; so effectively, in fact, that the appendix ruptured, abessed, and I then developed peritonitis. In those days any one of these was serious enough by itself; together they were frequently lethal. I was rushed to the hospital in Laurel for surgery; but, as my parents later related the incident, Dr. Gatlin emerged from the operating room to tell the family that I had died on the table—that I had no pulse, no respiration, dilated pupils, and that my body had turned "black as soot."

While our family was still together under one roof, this experience, together with comparable anecdotes about other members of the family, came to be among our most celebrated and treasured stories. When it was told, my mother would usually do the telling. Without all the embellishments that would obviously lend themselves to such a plot, the basic elements included: how the surgeon was asked whether there was any chance of resuscitation; how he answered no; how he was then asked to complete the operation because my mother did not want to bury her son with a gaping hole in his abdomen; how the surgeon then returned to the operating room to discover that I was somehow miraculously breathing again; and finally, how after nine months of bedridden convalescence I began, for the second time, to learn to walk.

I am told that what happened with my appendix thirty years ago is now a more or less routine procedure when compared with what doctors currently regard as a serious illness. And, despite the kinds of personal investment one understandably has in his own history, I have talked enough with doctors and surgeons and seen enough in hospital wards to be convinced that this is so. It is not that a ruptured, absessed appendix with the additional complication of peritonitis is no longer a serious illness; it is only that developed techniques and medications make this a more manageable illness than some others. But then that is how one would expect it to be in the history of medicine and its progressive movement toward the alleviation, and often cure, of human pain and disease.

Impressive new questions have been generated in the past three decades by the enormous strides of medicine and surgery. The issues which now confront us are considerably more complex and grave and awesome. Abortion, enlarging possibilities for controlling our genetic future, increased sensitivity toward human experimentation, organ transplantation, and the management of dying patients are only some of the profoundly perplexing as well as promising matters which urgently require sustained and serious attention from many competent people and a variety of perspectives. Indeed, I am convinced that there is perhaps greater need now than ever before for genuine interdisciplinary and interprofessional collaboration if we are to address these uniquely modern and deeply human concerns with integrity and responsibility.

One of the fictions which has contrived to prevent genuine interdisciplinary conversation between scientists and theologians maintains that science is *de*scriptive and that theology is *p*rescriptive. Or, as I have sometimes heard it said, scientists are question-askers and theologians are answer-givers; science describes the "is," while theology prescribes the "ought." That this kind of arbitrary, albeit neat, distinction is no longer tenable—if indeed it ever was—is one of the central assumptions of the chapters which follow. In fact, unless we are able to reconceive the parameters of useful conversation between science and theology on some ground other than their mutual exclusion, I think it self-evident that we cannot get very far beyond talking *about* one another. What we urgently must do, however—and there is almost daily evidence of both the need and the urgency of it—is learn to talk *with* each other.

I would not have ventured to write this book, I think, if this were not already happening and if my own experience with scientists and technologists, as well as theologians and ethicists, did not tend to confirm the view that interdisciplinary and inter-professional colleagueship is both increasingly necessary and increasingly possible. Among many reasons for this, two seem especially prominent to me. The acquisition and accumulation of knowledge is occurring at such an accelerated rate that it is difficult, if not frankly impossible, for a single discipline alone any longer to assimilate and apply its expertise responsibly to the full range of human affairs affected by it. The biological analogy may be that of neurologic overload. The second reason may be less obvious but I think no less valid: unlike earlier times when, in a struggle for their very existence, science and technology seemed often to be regarded by friend and foe alike as ends in themselves, I detect now a rather remarkable moral sensitivity among many scientists and technologists for the ends to which their knowledge and skills may be put. Concurrently, I sense a new kind of openness toward other disciplines and professions—an openness which not only tolerates well, but also actively solicits, mutuality and collaboration in matters of common human concern.

I know, of course, that these "reasons" are not universally demonstrable. Only recently at an international conference I listened to a British doctor who stated unequivocally that theologians are no longer of any help to physicians and surgeons (presumably they once were!), and that in consequence doctors themselves must formulate an "ethical code" which will satisfy the

11

majority of doctors and ensure both the well-being of individuals and the best interests of society. Meanwhile, he said, in a state of moral uncertainty and lack of precise moral direction, doctors must act according to their consciences.

There is in what this doctor said a certain evident truth; and it is that doctors must affirm their own values and do what they have to do. But there is also a certain deception in what he said; and that lies in the supposition that any profession which deals with persons, whether individually or societally, can insulate itself from competences of other humane disciplines and develop its own autonomous ethics. On the contrary, I wish to argue—and perhaps the conversation will be aided by putting it just this plainly—that there is no more urgent problem confronting the contemporary Christian ethicist than the tendency in some quarters to emancipate ethics from theology and to make decision-making processes autonomous and compartmentalized.

The basic premise of scientific and medical investigation is that underlying the immediate perplexity is a coherent whole. This is an assumption as dear to the moralist as it is to the natural scientist. And if this be granted and life characterized by purpose and intentionality rather than by whimsy and kismet, we are then relieved of the necessity to provide absolute and immutable answers to changing questions and free to offer provisional and tentative solutions which may do more to indicate the intentional direction of our existence than to resolve in some final way a given problematic.

There need be nothing strange or sinister about this holistic, intentional approach. If one describes a certain organism as being of such and such a character, having such and such chemical properties, and so on, and then claims that what has been said about that organism is a statement of what it is; then one has already also said in an implicit way what that organism is normatively—that is, what that organism must (or ought to) be in order to be that organism. One has already made a judgment about what ought to be in the process of describing what is. "Is" and "ought" may be appropriately differentiated, I do not doubt; but they need not therefore become the mutually exclusive references they have often been thought to be. We can distinguish without separating; and if this be granted, we may recover a holistic view of ourselves and our condition in which science and theology do not antagonize but rather complement each other.

To speak this way is not, of course, simply a matter of scientific deduction and proposition; it is also a judgment conditioned by culture and tradition. Thus another assumption which informs what follows is the notion that all who will read this book—doctors, lawyers, theologians, engineers, ethicists, and others—participate in a common heritage which makes us culturally *de facto* Judeo-Christians. I do not mean, to be sure, that all of us affirm the same doctrines or assent to the same creeds; the point is rather that, whatever our professed religious and ethical commitments, and however we formulate and express them privately, the kinds of questions being raised about what is important in modern biomedical technology, and how new data and skills are to be employed, could be raised only in a particular kind of culture which is (at least to the present time) dominated by the *de facto* operation of a particular view of man and the world which can be called Judeo-Christian. Thus what is the case with us already commits us to a discussion of what ought to be with us, and our decisions and choices are inescapably colored by that fact.

I therefore conceive the contribution of the professional theological ethicist to this discussion largely in terms of assessing and reflecting critically upon the human values at stake in medical decisions within the context of our shared *de facto* Judeo-Christian heritage. The ethicist's primary responsibility is not to provide answers, either gross or precise, but to help clarify and focus appropriate issues and problems and, in the measure to which it is fitting and desired, to participate in the adjudication of alternative choices and actions.

In one sense, it is rather a cruel joke to the ethicist's ego to discover that in situations like this he—like everyone else involved—is simply offering advice and making decisions in the light of his own best judgment and experience. In this respect he lays claim to no pre-eminent expertise. So while it makes sense to talk about practicing medicine or practicing law, there is no comparable sense in which we talk about practicing ethics as though this were a unique function of the ethicist which distinguishes

13

him from other people who practice other things! Nevertheless, given our increasing disciplinary and professional interdependency and our common *de facto* Judeo-Christian culture, perhaps it is arguable that the subtle and complex problems of modern human life need and deserve help, from whatever quarter.

I am deeply conscious in retrospect, as I was during the preparation of this book, of the assistance and encouragement of many persons. Among them are the "alumni" of two groups—the Medicine-Theology Group, based in Durham, North Carolina, and the Science-Theology Group, based in Raleigh—each of which, now reincarnated in other forms, amply demonstrated both the agony and the ecstasy of interdisciplinary dialogue. The extent of indebtedness to my students, both past and present, will be obvious only to them; so I need do no more than simply acknowledge it here. I also owe special thanks to the librarians of the Duke University Divinity School and the University of Edinburgh. Mrs. Vivian Crumpler and Mrs. Irma Gossett converted my untidy drafts into an orderly typescript. The index, always a painstaking task, has been admirably prepared by Miss Florence Russell.

Special grants in support of my research and writing were made by the American Association of Theological Schools, the Cooper Foundation, the Duke Endowment, and the Mary Biddle Duke Foundation. A travel grant was awarded by the Duke University Committee on International Studies. I gladly received this assistance, and now happily express my sincere thanks to those who made it possible for me.

I am indebted to a number of doctors who, in conversation over the years, have contributed to my medical education; and especially to Drs. Delford Stickel and Saul Boyarsky, whose friendship as well as professional competence I value highly. Professors Charles Curran, Louis Hodges, Paul Ramsey, and Charles Robinson were kind enough to read the manuscript and offer criticisms and suggestions. Among other friends and colleagues who have supported and encouraged my work in medicine and ethics, I want especially to acknowledge my thanks to Professors Joseph Fletcher, John Fletcher, and Donald Shriver.

Finally, to the women in my life—my wife and daughters, whose voices were "ever soft, gentle, and low; an excellent thing in woman"—I express a very special gratitude just for their being themselves.

There are doubtless some things still awry in this book, despite all the help for which I have just given thanks! But these will have to stand for just now. Meantime, in lieu of further apology, I will seek modest comfort from an old Southern aphorism: "It's no point in explainin'—your friends don't need it, and your enemies won't believe it anyway."

St. Luke's Day, 1970

I

Abortion and the Right to Life

In Western culture, pregnancy is thought of normatively as the fulfillment of a couple's cherished hope for children and family; when it occurs in this setting, all concerned welcome it as the realization of a deep natural instinct and the achievement of a genuine desire by this couple to concretize their one-flesh unity in human form. Whatever the pregnancy might signify to others, it is to those most immediately responsible for it a joyous event, a new life, their life in their baby, welcomed because it is wanted, and enjoyed because it proceeds uninterruptedly to term without serious complication.

But not every pregnancy conforms to this idealized pattern. Some are unplanned and unwanted; and others, although wanted and planned for, are threatened at some point by unexpected illness or disease or deformity which may affect either fetal or maternal health, or both. It is in these sorts of cases that the question of terminating pregnancy arises. But these conditions do not alone adequately indicate the complex problematics involved. Misleading oversimplification and confusion may perhaps be avoided if, at the very outset, we pay attention to the process which lies at the center of the abortion controversy and, in turn, identify the several indications which are commonly said to warrant the operation.

I

The beginning of life, like the end of it, is a process. At ejaculation the mature human male discharges approximately 250 to 300 million sperm cells, carrying paternal genetic information (DNA), into the vagina. From the vagina these sperm cells move through the uterus (womb) and into the fallopian tubes, where all of them will die in only a few days unless one unites with a viable egg. For her part, the mature human female ovulates once each month, and the egg thus produced, carrying maternal genetic information (DNA), passes from the ovary into the fallopian tubes on its way to the uterus (and usually expulsion in menstruation).

If the egg and sperm cells meet, one sperm cell may, though not necessarily, penetrate the egg, and when this occurs, fertilization has taken place. The newly fertilized egg, called a *zygote*, now combines both maternal and paternal genetic information and begins a journey of about six days through the fallopian tubes to the uterus. It is during this time that the fertilized egg starts the long and complex process of almost infinite cell division—from two cells to four, to eight, to sixteen, to thirty-two, and eventually to the billions of cells which constitute the human body. After six or seven days the *blastocyst*, as the tiny cluster of cells is now called, arrives in the uterus.

About 25 percent of all blastocysts are naturally expelled from the uterus in the monthly menstrual flow—a phenomenon which is described as "spontaneous abortion." If, however, a blastocyst is not naturally expelled or otherwise interfered with (as, for example, by drugs or mechanical devices), it has another six or seven days in which to implant itself in the membranous wall (the endometrium) of the uterus. This process is called *nidation*, and the cells which burrow into the uterine lining are called a *trophoblast*. One of the functions of the trophoblast is to signal the end of monthly menstruation. If this fails, the blastocyst is sloughed off and swept away in the menstrual flow, but if it succeeds, as it does

18

in 75 percent of cases, the trophoblast becomes the *placenta*, and its opposite pole (the blastocyst) becomes the *embryo*. The lapsed time from fertilization is about fourteen days.

After the second week following fertilization, there is rapid differentiation of certain organs—for example, brain, heart, liver; and by the end of six weeks the rudimentary development of all internal organs has normally taken place. It is common, from the eighth week, to refer to this nascent life as a *fetus*. At this time fingers and toes are recognizable, the skeleton takes form, the fetus has developed eyes but no eyelids, and simple reflex actions can be observed. No new major structures will be added to the organism; the remainder of its gestation period (approximately thirty weeks) will be spent in growth and maturation.

By the twelfth week bone and cartilage are clearly recognizable, the fetal heartbeat can be detected by electrocardiogram (EKG), and some movement may occur because of muscle and nerve development. The eyelids, nose, mouth, lips, ears, fingers, and toes are fully formed by the sixteenth week. If the fetus should for any reason spontaneously abort prior to the twentieth week, this natural expulsion is customarily called a miscarriage. After the twentieth week, such a natural expulsion of the fetus is referred to as premature birth. The period from the twentieth week to parturition (i.e., birth) is characterized by little change in the external appearance of the fetus, but internal organs (especially the brain, for example) undergo accelerated development. Viability of the fetus (i.e., its ability to live after birth) is ordinarily calculated from the beginning of the twenty-eighth week.[1] And if all else goes well, sometime around the 266th day since fertilization the zygote-blastocyst-trophoblast-embryo-fetus is delivered as a bouncing baby-boy-girl-infant-child.

Abortion is generally held to be safe for the woman if performed by qualified medical personnel under standard sterile operative conditions before the end of the twelfth week of gestation. To this point the standard procedure for abortion has been dilatation and

---

[1] Over the span from twenty to twenty-eight weeks the chance of fetal viability is calculated to be about 10 percent.

curettage.[2] More recently, vacuum aspiration of the conceptus is being increasingly employed both in this country and in Great Britain; a D&C is, however, still performed afterward.

It is during the first twelve weeks that the safety factor in abortion, under standard surgical conditions, is calculated in terms of minimal risk to maternal life and health. Moreover, it is also during these earlier stages of pregnancy that most of the symptoms currently recognized as indications of possible medical justification for abortion may manifest themselves.

There are, however, exceptions to this twelve-week rule: certain malformations or diseases which result in serious handicap to the fetus or present a grave risk to the mother do not become evident until very late in pregnancy, and sometimes only after birth. Anencephaly (absence of brain) and hydrocephaly (enlarged head caused by increased cerebral fluid), for example, are not liable to be diagnosed earlier than the thirty-second week. Certain hereditary conditions (Huntington's chorea, for example) are not detected until birth or later. Owing to these and other factors, it appears very unlikely that deformity and handicapping disease can be altogether eliminated from live births. It is also evident that an effort to eliminate as many defective fetuses as possible is (at least for the foreseeable future) bound to be generally restricted to the period after the first trimester. Meanwhile, the statistical probability is that one child in fifty births will present at least one serious defect of some sort.

Not all pregnancies, then, enjoy an uneventful course, and complicating factors which affect both fetal and maternal life do sometimes occur. But fetal and maternal lives are not the only ones affected by these events. The husband, other children, doctors, and many additional persons are more or less directly involved in a given pregnancy and its outcome. In the wider community of the human genetic pool there are all those—present and future—who will be more or less indirectly affected by decisions pertaining to a particular pregnancy. In consideration of these and other factors there are currently six discernible arguments which, in one situa-

[2] Dilatation and curettage is performed by stretching open the cervix, the narrow end of the uterus, and removing the conceptus with a scoop-shaped instrument called a curette.

tion or another, are defended as adequate justification for abortion. Not all of these arguments are universally advocated; neither are all of them explicitly sanctioned by law. All of them, however, have found proponents in recent debates, and we need now to indicate their principal features.

1. Some mothers-to-be encounter serious risk to their physical and/or mental health. If pregnancy under these conditions is permitted to go to term in these cases, there is real danger of damage to maternal health or loss of life. Cases in which there is irremediable conflict between nascent and maternal life are increasingly rare (now limited chiefly to serious renal or cardiac disease and certain well-defined mental diseases); nevertheless, the argument from maternal indications holds that serious risk to maternal health (mental and physical), as well as serious risk to maternal life, is adequate justification for abortion.

2. Some fetuses suffer a hereditary or genetic deformity; others may be abnormal or defective due to maternal disease or illness. We have already referred to Huntington's chorea as an example of a debilitating hereditary deformity. We can add, in this context, the crippling effects of a drug like thalidomide and the risks attendant on maternal exposure to rubella during the first trimester of pregnancy. Thousands of babies were born with congenitally deformed limbs and other defects as a direct result of their mothers' having taken the tranquilizing drug thalidomide. A significant number of these babies died of natural causes; though at least one, Corinne Van de Put—born with no arms, her face disfigured, and her anal canal emptying through her vagina—was killed by her mother.[3]

Exposure to rubella (infectious German measles) during the first twelve weeks of pregnancy carries at least a 50-50 risk that the infection will result in either (1) loss of the fetus through dangerous miscarriage, or (2) birth of a baby with one or more serious defects (mental retardation, blindness, heart defect, deafness, bone disease, or blood abnormality). As many as five such defects have been detected in a single affected child. A second

[3] Mrs. Suzanne Van de Put was subsequently tried for murder and acquitted. The jury in Liege, Belgium, agreed that Corinne had been *killed*, but not *murdered* (November, 1962).

argument in favor of abortion, then, is that certain pregnancies represent an inordinately high risk of fetal abnormality, and that consideration for both the family and the fetus indicate the preferability of not allowing this kind of pregnancy to proceed to term.

3. The social and eugenic consequences of rape and incest constitute a third argument for abortion. Neither rape nor incest accounts for large numbers of pregnancies, but when pregnancy does result from one of these actions, strong social feelings are aroused. There are both genetic and religious objections to incest, though many pregnancies which result from incest are allowed to come to term, and the baby is adopted. The objections to rape are more social and personal than scientific (except for the threat to maternal mental health that might accompany pregnancy as the result of rape). Some feel that if the mother-to-be does not want the child, she should not be made to bear it. Furthermore, it is sometimes argued that if the nascent life is hated by its bearer, the child will be brought forth into a situation devoid of love.

4. Experience demonstrates that a strong desire for an operation to be rid of an unwanted pregnancy can frequently be carried out, but often it must be conducted at considerable personal risk and outside conventional social and legal sanctions.

In 1967 the National Center for Health Statistics showed the birthrate at 17.9 per 1,000 population; numerically, about 3.5 million births. In the same year some experts were estimating that approximately one million abortions, 99 percent of them illegal, were being performed annually in the United States. Conversely, other experts argued that these figures were greatly inflated. Again in 1967 Dr. André Hellegers claimed that "about ten thousand therapeutic abortions are performed each year," and that "there are now about four hundred registered abortion deaths per year." Dr. Hellegers did not venture to estimate the number of *illegal* abortions performed annually, though he did (curiously) calculate that "it would be reasonable to assume that the annual number of deaths due to illegal abortions today might be on the general order of eight hundred or so *at most*." [4]

[4] André E. Hellegers, "Abortion, the Law, and the Common Good," *Medical Opinion and Review* (1967), 3:84, 90.

To this point the reliability of statistical data, together with their interpretation, is highly questionable. It is virtually impossible to confirm the accuracy of estimates because no way has yet been devised for obtaining exact figures for the total population. Neither can the number of alleged abortions be precisely correlated with specific reasons for seeking and obtaining abortion; nor is it particularly useful to project the number of deaths due to illegal abortion when this speculation is predicated upon the number of *registered* abortion deaths.

Whatever the precise statistics, there is enough evidence to warrant the observation that the demand for abortion in our society exceeds the legal, medical, and other provisions we have made for it. The consequence of this hiatus between demand and sanctioned auspices is the traffic in illegal abortion—a procedure which may involve infection, severe hemorrhage, future sterility, or death. The Kinsey Institute has reckoned that 20 to 25 percent of the white female population of the United States submit to illegal abortion sometime during their lives; and that the figure is comparable among upper-class Negro women but significantly higher among lower-class Negro women. In addition to those unfortunate women who die at the hands of illegal abortionists, thousands more suffer irreparable mutilations. The fourth argument for abortion claims that since a large number of abortions appear to be inevitable, it is preferable to provide adequate legal and therefore safer circumstances for their performance.

5. Some persons argue that abortion should be made available simply "on demand." Advocates of this view range from those who view abortion as an acceptable means for population control to the emergent radical feminists who argue that legal restraints are another evidence of the tyrannization of women in a repressive, male-dominated society. Neither of these groups is yet very prominent numerically, nor has either of them engendered large public support to date. Both, I think it fair to say, premise their arguments on utilitarian considerations which credit little or no regard to fetal life *qua se*. There is, nevertheless, a rather large latent constituency for both these points of view; and consideration of our present cultural situation tends to support the claim that their numbers will increase.

6. All the foregoing arguments have implied the final reason advanced in support of therapeutic abortion; and this is that the immediate threat to a wife and mother's health, or the long-range threat of having to rear a defective child, may make unreasonable demands on the existing family. It is far from clear, claim the proponents of this view, that an existing family ought to be sacrificed for a deformed fetus; rather, the converse is held to be true, and especially when there is a calculable statistical probability of serious fetal deformity or threat to maternal well-being.

II

Throughout the United States there are restrictive statutes which specify the conditions under which therapeutic abortion may be legally performed. Most states provide that if abortion is necessary to save the life or health of the mother, it is lawful; similarly, however, in many states statutes there is semantic ambiguity with respect to whether mental and emotional, as well as physical, well-being is an adequate criterion for legal abortion. In an effort to clarify these ambiguities and the consequent inequities under the law, the American Law Institute has put forward suggestions for uniform state statutes in its Model Penal Code. The ALI proposal provides that abortion *may* be legally elected when indicated by (1) substantial risk that continuation of the pregnancy would gravely impair the physical or mental health of the mother; (2) substantial risk that the child would be born with grave physical or mental defects; or (3) pregnancy which is the result of legally established rape or incest.[5]

Thirteen states (Alaska, Arkansas, California, Colorado, Delaware, Georgia, Hawaii, Kansas, Maryland, New Mexico, New York, North Carolina, and Oregon) have enacted legislation which incorporates some or all of the ALI proposals, and other states are in process of considering revision of existing statutes. Until there are uniform state statutes, the varying legal structures will continue to contribute to confusion and inequity before the law.

[5] *Model Penal Code*, Section 230.3(2), (3). Proposed Official Draft, 1962.

There are those who argue that all abortion statutes should be abolished on the premise that abortion statutes are either unconstitutional or else too vaguely worded and ambiguous to guarantee justice under the law. Their shared assumption is that abortion is a *private* matter between a pregnant woman and a physician professionally competent to perform this operation. I do not altogether agree with this view; moreover, I find Paul Ramsey's comment on the law's interest in abortion to be both cogent and faithful to the facts:

The legal reason for prohibiting abortion is not because it is believed to be a species of murder; it is the religious tradition . . . and not the law which inculcates the latter view. The law's presumption is only that society has a stake in the prehuman material out of which the unique individual is to be born. Or it may be that the law exhibits a belief that as a matter of public policy society has an interest in *men* and *women*, who have an interest in and by their actions take responsibility for the prehuman material out of which an individual human being is to be brought forth a man alive.[6]

It is of utmost importance to understand that *none of the current arguments or legislative bills makes abortion mandatory; they are instead permissive throughout.* Of course, "permissive" does not (and cannot, in the nature of the case) imply the complete absence of coercion; indeed, a question of abortion would not arise if there were not strong and persistent pressures to consider it as an option. It deserves frank acknowledgment, moreover, that even permissive laws yield additional moral pressure— that is, the pedagogy of the law sometimes leads people to conclude that because an action is legal, it must (generally, at least, in these sorts of cases) be right. Still, it would be neither fair nor correct to argue that proposals for statutory reform are only thinly disguised mechanisms for population control or the alleviation of economic problems for a family.

At the pragmatic level of administering the law in the interests of justice, however, my strong and increasingly confirmed opinion

---

[6] Paul Ramsey, "The Morality of Abortion," in Daniel H. Labby, ed., *Life or Death: Ethics and Options* (Seattle: University of Washington Press, 1968), pp. 64-65.

is that all the current abortion statutes (the recently revised, as well as the older laws) do discriminate operationally against a pregnant woman's freedom to elect abortion. This is especially true in the measure to which medical examiners exercise determinative judgments in the decision-making process. There is more than ample evidence that medical certification for legal abortions is highly variable, that it is very difficult to secure certification from some doctors and, conversely, very easy to obtain it from some others. There is much, of course, that is at stake in consideration of abortion; but the woman's right, in a free society, to make the ultimate decision—however much informed by medical, moral, and other opinion—surely should be among the highest priorities and deserves safeguarding.

All the arguments and indications currently being advanced presuppose certain informing principles, which in turn raise important questions: Is it true that maternal and/or other mature life ought sometimes to be preferred to nascent life? that all lives of the human species are not equal? that some lives are worth more than others or at least enjoy a certain priority? that universal laws may sometimes be modified by extenuating circumstances? In addition, there is also a certain relationship between socio-legal warrants for procedures of this sort and our own ideals for self-determination and individual liberty. In order to examine some of these assumptions more closely and perceive how they have come to be a part of our common life, we must now look briefly at the history of theological speculation in the Christian West on the question of the inviolability of human species life. And in the process of doing this, we can proceed to test the adequacy of both the arguments which favor abortion and the conventional Christian wisdom which often opposes it.

III

The earliest abortifacient recipe is thought to be over 4,500 years old, and it is well known that induced abortion was employed as a mechanism for birth control long before the Christian era. Indeed, infanticide was widely practiced among both Greeks and Romans for purposes of population control. Such legal restraints as there were, however, existed not for the protection of nascent life but (1) for the safeguarding of maternal life (because many women died as the direct result of primitive abortion techniques), and (2) for guaranteeing that husbands would not be deprived of children by wives who were vain, or fearful, or otherwise unwilling to become mothers.

Initial Christian objection to abortion, and also to infanticide, was grounded in speculation about the soul—its origin, its existence in time, and its ultimate destiny. The Greeks had similarly developed notions about the soul as an eternal and indestructible part of the total human being. Despite this fact both Aristotle and Plato sanctioned (and, on occasion, encouraged) abortion. Perhaps it was the Christian doctrine of divine sovereignty—that as the beginning and continuation of creation is God's work, so also must be its end—that eventually swung the balance in Western civilization. In any case, Greek sanction for abortion as an instance of human mastery over the Real in its struggle toward the Ideal gave way to Christian prohibition of abortion on the principle of inviolability of human soul-formed life, whose beginning and end involves an act of God.

At least three different theories of the origin of the soul and the time of its union with the body have been held in Western Christendom. (1) Tertullian, representing *traducianism* or *generationism*, held that the soul (*anima*) came into existence with the body as a biological transmission from Adam through one's immediate parents.[7] Not only was fiat creation reaffirmed by this teaching, but in addition, the way was prepared for the doctrine of inherited original sin. (2) Clement of Alexandria, on the other hand, held that the soul was immediately and directly created by God. This view, understandably, is called *creationism.*[8] (3) The third position claimed that no soul was present in fetal life until the moment of "quickening," that moment when the mother-to-be detected the first stirrings of life within her body. Augustine

[7] Tertullian, "De Anima," 27, in J.-P. Migne, ed., *Patrologiae Cursus Completus,* Series Latina (Parisii: Apud Garnier Fratres, 1879), II, 694.

[8] Clement of Alexandria, "Stromata," IV, 6, in Alexander Roberts and James Donaldson, eds., *The Ante-Nicene Fathers* (Grand Rapids: Eerdmans Publishing Co., 1951), II, 413-16.

27

of Hippo, an advocate of this view, was suspicious of both crea-tionist and generationist arguments. Against the creationists, he maintained that the Bible does not offer conclusive proof that the soul is directly and immediately created by God. Moreover, he added that in view of the stain of original sin upon the soul, one ought to be cautious about attributing direct creation to God! His controversy with the Pelagians, on the other hand, made him suspicious of concluding that the soul comes into being by nat-ural generation.[9]

By the Middle Ages no definitive position had been generally accepted; and it was Thomas Aquinas, influenced by interpretive clues from the Mediterranean world as well as by Christian spec-ulators, who formulated the predominant medieval view that the soul is not created at conception, but at the time when it is "infused" into the body. He reckoned this "infusion" to occur at about the fortieth day in the male embryo and at about the eightieth day in the female embryo.[10]

IV

It was not until the seventeenth century, in fact, that current Roman Catholic doctrine on the inviolability of nascent life began to take definite doctrinal shape. In his 1679 decree, *Errores doctrinae moralix laxioris*, Pope Innocent XI maintained (1) that it is illicit to induce abortion before animation in order to spare a pregnant girl death or shame, (2) that it is erroneous doctrine that every fetus lacks a rational soul so long as it con-fined to the womb and only begins to have a soul at the time it is born, and (3) that it is prohibited to hold any longer "that

---

[9] Augustine, "De Anima et ejus Origine," in Philip Schaff, ed., A *Select Library of the Nicene and Post-Nicene Fathers of the Christian Church* (Grand Rapids: Eerdmans Publishing Co., 1956), V, 315-71. Cf. Augustine, "Ad. Optat." 190, al. 157, in Migne, *Patrologiae Cursus Completus*, Series Latina, XXXIII, 861.

[10] Thomas Aquinas, *Summa Theologica*, trans. Fathers of the English Dominican Province (New York: Benziger Brothers, 1947), Part I, q. 118, arts. 1-3. See also *De animalibus*, IX, or *De generatione animalium*.

no homicide is committed in any abortion." [11] As is often the case in the evolution of theological doctrine, Innocent XI's decree did not promulgate a specific and positive teaching so much as it merely condemned certain erroneous views. Regarding the time of animation, Fr. Gerald Kelly rightly says that "we have no divine revelation on this point, nor any official pronouncement of the Church which clearly condemns or approves either theory." [12]

Still, Roman Catholicism has come to a developed position on the question of abortion, and it deserves to be acknowledged: *practically we should act as if we knew* that the soul is infused at conception. And the reason for this, as I perceive it, is that theoretical uncertainty in so important a matter as the right to life deserves to be resolved into practical certainty. Fr. Bernard Häring thus accurately reflects the position of modern Roman Catholicism when he states that "today the view that the soul is infused immediately at the moment of conception is almost universally accepted by physicians, and especially by theologians." [13]

Pope Pius XI, in his 1930 encyclical *Casti Connubii*, maintained the inviolability of fetal life on the grounds that it is "equally sacred" with the life of the mother, and he described medical and therapeutic indications for abortion as excusing "the direct murder of the innocent." More to the point, Canon 747 insists that "every aborted fetus shall be baptized without any condition, if it is known with certainty that it is alive, no matter at what period of gestation it is aborted; if there is doubt that it is alive, it shall be baptized conditionally. *The obligation imposed extends to even the smallest fetus, even though it be aborted immediately after conception.*" [14]

---

[11] Henricus Denzinger, *Enchiridion Symbolorum: Definitionum et Declarationum de Rebus Fidei et Morum* (32nd ed. rev.; Freiburg im Breisgau: Verlag Herder KG, 1963), p. 461.

[12] Gerald Kelly, *Medico-Moral Problems* (St. Louis: The Catholic Hospital Association of the United States and Canada, 1958), p. 66.

[13] Cf. Bernard Häring, *The Law of Christ* (Paramus, N. J.: Paulist-Newman Press, 1966), III, 205. For arguments in favor of later animation, see Joseph Donceel, "Abortion: Mediate v. Immediate Animation," *Continuum* (1967), 5:167-71.

[14] John A. Abbo and Jerome D. Hannan, *The Sacred Canons* (St. Louis: B. Herder Book Co., 1952), I, 752-53. Italics added.

Both *Casti Connubii* and Canon 747 employ inference and oblique commentary, but the intended teaching is unmistakable in both. Given the sacramental theology of Roman Catholicism, and the notion of baptismal regeneration in particular, Canon 747 clearly supposes that an eternal but original-sin-tainted soul is present from the moment of fertilization; and all the elaborate provisions for guaranteeing fetal baptism, whether *in* or *ex utero*, further support the notion that unbaptized nascent life is in spiritual jeopardy.

Moral theologians and popular directives have been less evasive. Fr. Charles McFadden puts the point succinctly, if rather bluntly: "Direct and voluntary abortion is a moral offense of the gravest nature, since it is the deliberate destruction of an innocent life. . . . Such an action is essentially murder." [15] Fr. Eberhard Welty agrees: "At the moment when conception occurs in the mother's womb, God infuses the soul and human life begins. . . . To kill this helpless creature with full knowledge and free consent is to commit murder. This argument admits of no exception." [16] And the *Ethical and Religious Directives for Catholic Hospitals* states unequivocally in directive 14: "Every unborn child must be regarded as a human person, with all the rights of a human person, from the moment of conception." [17]

In practice the Catholic prohibition against abortion is modified by an important adjective, namely, *direct*. From this exception certain interesting qualifications follow. What is prohibited, *ubique semper et ab omnibus*, is direct abortion; that is, an action which has as its primary thrust a deliberate attempt to kill the fetus or incapacitate it in such a way that it is likely to die. Direct abortion is always prohibited on the ground that maternal and fetal life are equal, and therefore neither may licitly be preferred to the other.

[15] Charles J. McFadden, *Medical Ethics* (5th ed. rev.; Philadelphia: F. A. Davis Co., 1961), p. 132.

[16] Eberhard Welty, *A Handbook of Christian Social Ethics* (Freiburg: Herder & Herder, 1953), II, 123.

[17] *Ethical and Religious Directives for Catholic Hospitals* (2nd. ed. rev.; St. Louis: The Catholic Hospital Association of the United States and Canada, 1957).

But indirect abortion, as Catholic moralists testify, is another matter. Indirect abortion occurs when an action has the *secondary* effect of expelling or destroying the fetus *in utero*, and is justified under the rule (or principle) of double effect. This rule eventuates from a formula which supposes that an action might produce two effects: one of which is good and intended, and the other of which is evil and unintended but inevitable. Four specific conditions, however, must be fulfilled in order to employ this principle: (1) the action, considered by itself and independently of its effects, must not be morally evil; (2) the evil effect must not be the means of producing the good effect; (3) the evil effect is merely tolerated and sincerely *un*intended; (4) there must be a proportionate reason for performing the action despite its evil consequences. Indirect abortion is supposed to be just such an action.

"Thus," says Fr. Henry Davis, "if a mother is in serious danger of death, she may take medicines or submit to treatment on herself necessary for her recovery and directly conducive to it even if, at the same time, the fetus is ejected or dies *in utero*, provided that it is guarded against as far as possible, and that nothing is done to induce it directly, i.e., by direct action on the fetus." [18] In other words, an action which has as its primary thrust and intention the saving of maternal life may be employed under the rule of double effect, even though the consequence of this action entails the certain (but unintended) death of nascent life. In a specific case, for example, a hysterectomy may be performed for malignant ovarian tumor even when a pregnant uterus is involved. Focusing on the primacy of intention, it is supposed, permits the morality of an action to be shifted from considerations of personal responsibility and liability to elaborations of excuses for existential or some other necessity.[19]

[18] Henry Davis, *Moral and Pastoral Theology* (5th ed. rev.; London: Sheed and Ward, 1946), II, 169.

[19] Although our primary concern here is to describe the official and predominating teaching of Roman Catholicism, it deserves notice that some Catholic moralists are themselves criticizing the conventional distinctions between direct and indirect actions. Fr. Charles Curran, for example, argues that the customary understanding of direct and indirect "is inadequate precisely because of a tendency to identify the human action in terms of the physical structure of the action. . . . I do not think that the ultimate moral decision

An additional and similar qualification has to do with the provisions under which Catholic doctors and nurses may licitly participate in surgical abortions. Under the distinction between direct and indirect actions one may further discriminate between formal and material types of cooperation, which are defined by a prominent Catholic jurist as follows:

Formal cooperation . . . occurs when one acts with another in performing an external act which is wrong in itself with or without internal assent, or where assistance is given to one performing an immoral act by an act in itself indifferent but with the intention of promoting the evil action. Material cooperation is the performance of an indifferent act helping another's evil act but with no intention of forwarding it.[20]

Catholic doctors and nurses may licitly participate in surgical abortions, then, if they do so only materially and for a serious reason (for example, grave inconvenience to the surgical team or definite threat to one's professional future). These conditions being satisfied, however, a Catholic doctor could presumably serve as anesthetist, and a Catholic nurse could scrub to assist the surgeon performing an abortion.

These are subtle and fine points to grasp; perhaps, in the final analysis, too subtle and fine to be of much practical help in decision-making. Not only are they worrisome in their microscopic attention to self-conscious differences between intentions and actions, but few of the situations which might, even in theory, warrant this kind of moral precision would appear to afford sufficient leisure—before, during, or often even after the act—for such exhaustive analysis of superfine facets of one's exact intentions and actions. Beyond this obvious difficulty, the human psyche has its own ways of rationalizing necessity and complicity.

---

in complex circumstances can be decided on the basis of the physical structure of an action and the sole, immediate, physical effect of an action. All the moral values must be considered and a final decision made after all the moral values have been compared." (Cf. Curran, *A New Look at Christian Morality* [Notre Dame, Ind.: Fides Publishers, 1968], pp. 237-43; pp. 238-39 quoted.)

[20] Norman St. John-Stevas, *Life, Death and the Law* (Bloomington: Indiana University Press, 1961), p. 195.

In the end one may wonder whether these circumlocuitous propositions are functionally worth the time and effort required to apply them in a particular instance. In fact, it is precisely this kind of anticipation and prescription for every imaginable sort of exigency that has given casuistry (whether Catholic or Protestant) a bad name as a synonym for legalism.

Perhaps we can illustrate the inadequacy of arguing double effects and direct/indirect distinctions at the pragmatic level of decision-making by referring again to sterilization as a procedure which is, in certain ways, corollary to abortion. It would never be ecclesiastically lawful for a Catholic doctor to perform direct sterilization under any circumstance, although he might give material cooperation or effect sterilization indirectly by performing, for example, hysterectomy for malignant ovarian tumor. He is similarly prohibited from performing direct abortion under any circumstances, although he might also give material cooperation or excise a pregnant uterus in the process, for example, of performing hysterectomy for malignant ovarian tumor.

The functional muddle which eventuates from this moral posture is indicated by the following propositions: direct sterilization is not permitted, even in order to prevent pregnancy in a woman who is herself so diseased that a pregnancy will directly endanger her life and that of the fetus; *during pregnancy*, however, both abortion and sterilization may be licitly performed (i.e., indirectly) if necessary to save the woman's life!

The strengths of the Roman Catholic approach to abortion are principally twofold. First, throughout the entire discussion of abortion there is conviction that God's will for the conduct of human life, even in borderline situations, is well enough known so that no person need feel bereft of divine guidance or solely dependent upon his own private sense of right and wrong. Second, there is the frank recognition that where duties, obligations, and rights are not authoritatively defined but left solely to the private judgment of each individual, we are only a step away from anarchic decisions which are morally intolerable.

But what remains at issue parallels these strengths. Methodologically, it is arguable that the morphology and character of

33

God's will and the moral guidance it provides are rather more open to relativity, provisionality, and experimentation than a rigid and doctrinaire correlation between natural law and divine intention acknowledges. Pragmatically, a conceptualization of "human" in relational rather than substantive terms affords an openness to existential novelty and innovation by refusing (or being unable!) to predefine in every not-yet instance the precise shape and fit of personal responsibility.

Despite emphasis on the distinctly human elements in decision-making—for example, on intention as this affects indirect action or material cooperation—Catholic pronouncements nevertheless tend to vitiate human judgment by insisting upon rightness or wrongness as *intrinsic* qualities of certain actions.

Pope Pius XI's encyclical, *Casti Connubii*, illustrates the rigidity and confirms distrust of such an objectivizing approach. Referring to the medical and therapeutic indications for abortion, the Pope reasoned that concern and pity for a pregnant woman whose health and even life is gravely imperiled by threatening fetal life cannot excuse her or us from "the duty allotted to her by nature." And Fr. McFadden, echoing the judgment of this encyclical, has translated the papal rhetoric into a harsh maxim: "No matter how readily and certainly direct abortion could preserve a mother's life or health, it is not morally permissible. . . . It is nothing more or less than the deliberate murder of an innocent life in order to preserve thereby the life or health of the mother." [21] Such rigorism in ethics, extrapolated from a certain kind of natural law theory, both depersonalizes and dehumanizes the decision-making process, and finally subordinates man's capacity (however limited) for self-determination and purpose to the erratic, sometimes capricious, but always impersonal forces of his natural environment.

[21] McFadden, *Medical Ethics*, p. 135. It was indicated earlier that some Catholic moralists are raising serious questions regarding the sufficiency of such statements as this. And if one takes seriously the ecumenical spirit that seems increasingly to inform Catholic-Protestant dialogue, it may not be unreasonable to hope that the division between Catholic and Protestant as such on these and similar issues will give way to more adequate formulations by both sides.

V

An examination of representative statements from Protestant spokesmen is, almost by definition, a much more diffuse undertaking than the comparable task with Roman Catholics. Indeed, Dean Fitch's analysis of internal tensions in these two branches of Christendom is altogether apposite here: "There is a Catholic strength, and its name is order. There is a Catholic sickness, and its name is tyranny. There is a Protestant strength, and its name is liberty. There is a Protestant sickness, and its name is anarchy." [22] Notwithstanding the force of this observation, even a cursory look will remind us that as among Catholics there are exceptions to rules and conscientious limits to tyranny, so among Protestants there are boundaries to liberty and dykes against anarchy. Our major difficulty here is that so few Protestant theologians have ventured to address themselves seriously to medical and bio-medical questions.

Helmut Thielicke has argued that the sanctity of human species life, and therefore its inviolability, is established at fertilization: "Once impregnation has taken place, it is no longer a question of whether the persons concerned have responsibility for a *possible* parenthood; they have *become* parents." On the very next page, however, Thielicke defends the inviolability of nascent human life by the claim that "the fetus has its own autonomous life. . . . The fetus has its own circulatory system and its own brain. The elementary biological fact should be sufficient to establish its status as a human being." [23] But this is a biological development, as we have seen, that does not occur in even a rudimentary fashion until sometime between the second and sixth weeks' post-fertilization. Perhaps the most generous construction that might be placed on Thielicke's claim about "autonomous life" would seek to construe that expression as referring to the value of nascent life vis-à-vis maternal (and presumably other) life which impinges upon it; but the context clearly fails to support this interpretation.

[22] Robert E. Fitch, "The Protestant Sickness," *Religion in Life* (1966), 35:498-505.
[23] Helmut Thielicke, *The Ethics of Sex*, trans. John W. Doberstein (New York: Harper & Row, 1964), pp. 227, 228.

Instead, Thielicke seems to be speaking of a *biologically* conditioned status, claiming that because the fetus has its own circulatory system and brain, it is autonomous. No commonsense definition of "autonomous," however, will support its use to describe the biological status of either zygote, embryo, or fetus. As we saw earlier, a fetus is regarded as viable from the twenty-eighth week of pregnancy; fetuses delivered prior to this time rarely survive. But beyond that present fact, fetuses are not autonomous in any precise meaning of that word—even after 266 days of gestation! Nor, for that matter, are human beings—at any point between life and death—ever "independent" or autonomous except in a profoundly contingent and comparative sense.

Thielicke's reasons for attributing *humanitas* to zygote or embryo appear to be formally those of Roman Catholicism (i.e., naturalistic at base), and his misinformation (or perhaps uncertainty) about prenatal processes is taken to confirm an otherwise independently formulated speculation. Nevertheless, Thielicke does not follow the inexorable logic of Catholic casuistry in this matter. Instead, he entertains the possibility of therapeutic abortion by arguing that we live in the "order of *necessity* in the fallen world," and that "what we see in the world as disorder can never be related directly to God's creatorhood and his government of the world." Indeed, war and sickness and suffering are cited as illustrations of the fact that "it is not God's *real* will that is at work in the perversity of the world." [24]

Thielicke has correctly pointed here to an incommensurability between God's perfect will and the options and alternatives which are available to us in historical decision-making crises. He observes that we cannot venture to decide certain questions (for example, irremediable conflict between two lives) with "precise theological exactitude." He cannot, however, bring himself to face squarely the issues raised by direct therapeutic abortion. Instead, he talks around the central question: "In the borderline situation the overwhelming force of these questions . . . brings out very clearly what is always the case, namely, that we can decide only subject to forgiveness," and, "Obviously there is a difference between the rela-

[24] *Ibid.*, p. 237. Italics added.

tionship which we have with a living person and that which we have with a human life which is beginning to germinate." [25] Thus he curiously evades a straightforward encounter with the issues.

There is surely no doubt that Christians always act subject to forgiveness; and there may even be general agreement that relationships are different with pre- and post-natal species life. But what does this kind of language mean, apart from arguing for some relative freedom in decision-making and acknowledging that human relationships vary in perceived intensity and range? On the premise that the emergency orders by which God preserves a fallen world sometimes allow (or constrain) one to take life, it *may* be the excusability—but not justification—of abortion that Thielicke is arguing for. In the end, however, he does not say precisely what the difference in relationships is, but merely that the "widespread feeling" that embryonic life is "only a part of the maternal organism, and that in the case of conflict the whole takes precedence over the part" is wrong! [26] It seems to me reasonable to contend that if there is an important difference, we need, and are entitled, to know what it is.

His final comment simply reaffirms his initial claims: (1) "We point to the plain biological fact that the embryo has its own autonomy, on the basis of which the germinating life must be interpreted as the developing of a *humanitas* which is already there," and (2) "The fact that the diminutive embryo is actually human life and therefore just as sacrosanct as any human life remains beyond question." [27]

Thielicke suggests a reformulation of the dualistic approach to decision-making. Such a construction is especially intimated by the polarization of (1) absolute certainty that nascent species life is inviolable and sacrosanct and (2) affirmation of mundane disorder which illustrates only or chiefly the absence of God's "real will" in human affairs. Privately and personally, one is presumably called upon to honor and protect prenatal species life as an evidence of God's creatorhood in and through natural pro-

[25] *Ibid.*, pp. 242, 243.
[26] *Ibid.*, p. 244.
[27] *Ibid.*, pp. 244, 245.

37

cesses; in public and official capacities, however, one is free to make onerous choices between lives equally human because he is assured that "it is not God's *real* will that is at work in the perversity of the world." [28]

But this, as students of theological ethics know, begs the question of human responsibility for human acts. In addition, Thielicke leaves the unfortunate (and unwarranted) impression that the only God we perceive in historically conditioned decision-crises is the *Deus absconditus*. We still need a theological approach to the question, "What makes life human?"

Dietrich Bonhoeffer is well known as the promising young theologian who was hanged by the Nazis in 1944 and as the author of *The Cost of Discipleship* and *Letters and Papers from Prison.* But it is his posthumously published and unfinished *Ethics* that most directly concerns us here. In his brief section on "Reproduction and Nascent Life," Bonhoeffer argues (1) that the embryo's existence is itself evidence of God's intention to create a human being, (2) that the embryo's right to life is therefore divinely bestowed, and (3) that any deliberate deprivation of it is "nothing but murder." [29] If one asks whether embryonic life is already human or not, Bonhoeffer's response is that such a question as this merely confuses the issue.

Indeed, the relationship between divine intention and nascent inviolability is so pervasive in Bonhoeffer's thought that it "backs up," as it were, into the marriage covenant itself. Unless a couple acknowledges the sacred right-to-be of life that is to come into being, their marriage "ceases to be marriage and becomes a mere liaison." Moreover, a marriage in which the desire for children is consistently excluded or denied is a "contradiction to the meaning of marriage itself." [30] On Bonhoeffer's terms couples apparently have no choice about *whether* to have children; their only options are *when* and *how many!*

Finally, on the question of irremediable conflict between nascent and maternal life, Bonhoeffer is again unswerving in his

[28] *Ibid.*, p. 237.
[29] Dietrich Bonhoeffer, *Ethics*, trans. N. H. Smith (New York: The Macmillan Co., 1955), p. 131.
[30] *Ibid.*, pp. 130, 131.

deference to the life-that-is-to-come-into-being. In a footnote to the paragraph which includes the key sentence, "Destruction of the embryo in the mother's womb is a violation of the right to live which God has bestowed upon this nascent life," Bonhoeffer simply marks off from human competence the matter of choosing between nascent and maternal life: "The life of the mother is in the hand of God," he concludes, "but the life of the child is arbitrarily extinguished." [31]

Despite emphasis on divine intention as the criterion for pre-natal inviolability, Bonhoeffer, like Thielicke, adopted a kind of naturalistic referent for determining the way out of the terrible choice. Whatever is developing—in however arrested or potential a stage of development—is in itself sufficient evidence that God intends for it to come into being.

To locate the principle of inviolability in the divine will is, I think, an appropriate step, but Bonhoeffer has quite mistakenly described God's will as merely a postulate inferred from observation of nature.[32] It is far from clear, for example, on what other grounds he maintains that nascent life should tyrannize maternal life when the two are irreconcilably in conflict. Indeed, what Bonhoeffer asks and advocates is that we abandon responsibility for direct decision in this situation, on the apparent assumption that nature's way is God's way. But this is an impotent *moral* posture as well as an untenable basis for medical practice. We can no more forego direct and intentional interference with natural processes than we can abdicate human moral judgments to an insensitive fatalism.

On the other side of the Protestant spectrum, Joseph Fletcher has argued that the basic problem of those who oppose direct abortion is their commitment to a position "which attributes personal status to a pre-personal organism and assigns it human rights." The way out of this dilemma, according to Fletcher, is relatively uncomplicated: deny the validity of the right to life

---

[31] *Ibid.*

[32] This tendency can be appreciated (historically, at least) if one recalls that Schweitzerian romanticism was widespread among theologians in the 1930's. Cf. Albert Schweitzer, "The Ethics of Reverence for Life," *Christendom* (1936), 1:225-29.

claimed for nascent organisms on the grounds that "a fetus is not a moral or personal being since it lacks freedom, self-determination, rationality, the ability to choose either means or ends, and knowledge of its circumstances." In Fletcher's opinion the embryo before birth is only a "portion of the mother, which may be excised if it threatens her life" on the principle that it is licit to sacrifice a part for the sake of the whole.[33]

Because Fletcher's discussion of abortion occurs as a brief excursus in a chapter titled "Sterilization: Our Right to Foreclose Parenthood," it unfortunately fails to give detailed response to the naturalistic position against which Fletcher's personalism claims to stand. There is no doubt, however, that Fletcher explicitly rejects consideration of a supernatural soul as a criterion which might assign inviolability to nascent life, or even as a possible factor which might pose a serious dilemma for moral decision-making: "We put the priority on personality, and frankly view with skepticism the claim for a soul as an entity apart from life and personal being." [34]

Similarly, he has no apparent intention of reducing the human dimension (however that may be described) to a merely biological mechanism (of whatever sort). Nor is there any indication in Fletcher's work that inviolability as such attaches absolutely to any kind of life which cannot be said, on his definition, to be "moral and personal." The anxiety which is generated by this approach does not lie in the precision and rigidity of antecedently fixed rules, according to Fletcher, but in the question of who is going to decide when freedom, self-determination, and all the rest are sufficiently present in a given instance of species life to guarantee its sanctity.

It is to Fletcher's credit that he rejects fertilization or any other fixed biological point as definitive of whatever it means to be human and personal; indeed, the deep humanism which pervades his writing is commendable if for no other reason than that it offers one of the few modern alternatives to the absolutist and intrinsicalist ethics of conventional religion. His is a deliberate

---

[33] Joseph Fletcher, *Morals and Medicine* (Boston: Beacon Press, 1960), pp. 150, 152.

[34] *Ibid.*, p. 163.

effort to humanize decision-making so that persons may become increasingly responsible for control of their historical existence and destiny.

On the other hand, some of the questions he so summarily answers deserve significantly more probing analysis and careful attention (for example, whether embryonic life is, after all, merely a dispensable portion of the maternal whole). In sum, Fletcher has greatly oversimplified what are, in fact, profoundly complex matters, and in the process presented an exaggeratedly optimistic anthropology. One of the clues that prompts this judgment lies in the relative disregard which Fletcher holds for nascent life. Saying this, I do not mean to suggest, of course, that he holds or advocates strong negative feelings toward fetal life, but only that he tends, in my judgment, to regard and treat it more casually than it deserves.[35]

Paul Ramsey has produced an assortment of probing and perceptive ethical analyses on a wide variety of subjects. We need refer to only two of them here in order to review in an admittedly too-brief synopsis the approach of a Protestant moralist who takes seriously the relevance of natural law theory for Christian ethics.

In an article titled "The Sanctity of Life," [36] Ramsey devoted several pages to elucidating the distinctions and theories regarding when germinating life becomes human, before concluding that

[35] The stated premise of the chapter in which Fletcher discusses abortion is a quotation from the 1930 White House Conference on Child Health and Protection: "There should be no child in America that has not the complete *birthright* of a sound mind in a sound body, and that has not been born under proper conditions." (*Ibid.*, p. 141.) This is a praiseworthy ambition, no doubt, but not without its own great (who is to say whether too great?) cost, as Norman St. John-Stevas illustrates: "Maurice Baring used to tell the following story. One doctor to another: 'About the terminating of a pregnancy, I want your opinion. The father was syphilitic. The mother tuberculous. Of the four children born, the first was blind, the second died, the third was deaf and dumb, the fourth also tuberculous. What would you have done?' 'I would have ended the pregnancy.' 'Then you would have murdered Beethoven.'" (Norman St. John-Stevas, *The Right to Life* [New York: Holt, Rinehart & Winston, 1963], p. 16.)

[36] Paul Ramsey, "The Sanctity of Life," *The Dublin Review* (1967), 241:3-23. This article, slightly emended but substantially unchanged, subsequently appeared as a chapter in a symposium. Cf. Paul Ramsey, "The Morality of Abortion," *Life or Death: Ethics and Options*, pp. 60-93.

41

"from an authentic religious point of view none of them matters very much." The reason for this rather abrupt announcement is that the question of *when* sanctity attaches to human life is not religiously problematic at all: "One grasps the religious outlook upon the sanctity of human life only if one sees that this life is asserted to be *surrounded* by sanctity that need not be in a man; that the most dignity a man ever possesses is a dignity that is alien to him. . . . A man's dignity arises from God's dealings with him, and not primarily in anticipation of anything he will ever have it in him to be." [37] From this perspective, Ramsey argues, it is relatively unimportant to establish *when*, along the continuum of species life, we are or are not dealing with a life that is human.

This emphasis on God's value for life, which we encountered earlier in Bonhoeffer, is reinforced in later sections of the same article:

The value of a human life is ultimately grounded in the value God is placing on it. . . . [Man's] sacredness is not composed by observable degrees of relative worth. A life's sanctity consists not in its worth *to* anybody . . . . No one is ever much more than a fellow fetus; and in order not to become confused about life's primary value it is best not to concentrate on degrees of relative worth we may later acquire. . . . [Man's] essence is his existence before God and to God, as it is from him. His dignity is "an *alien* dignity; an evaluation that is not of him but placed upon him by the divine decree." [38]

The practical consequence of all this, as Ramsey interprets it, is that every human being, at whatever stage of his becoming this kind of being, is surrounded by protections and prohibitions which assert the sanctity of human life. We are all fellow fetuses together, and distinctions between us are wholly relative. Because our value is God's valuation of us, any direct action which violates the naked equality of one life with another is prohibited. On this ground Ramsey supports the Roman Catholic distinction between direct and indirect abortion and argues that in cases of irremediable conflict between nascent and maternal lives (i.e., a conflict of equals) only *indirect* abortion is morally licit. "This

[37] "The Sanctity of Life," pp. 9-10.
[38] *Ibid.*, pp. 10-11.

rule of moral practice," he says, "seems to be both a logical and a charitable extension of ethical deliberations impelled by respect for the *equal* sanctity of both the lives that are in mortal conflict and both of whom one wants to save." [39]

The only exception to this rule, according to Ramsey, occurs in those situations, however rare, in which *both* nascent and maternal lives will be forfeit unless action is taken to kill the fetus. In this circumstance, "it is permissible, nay, it is even morally obligatory, to kill the fetus directly if, without this, both mother and child will die together." But even under these extenuating conditions, Ramsey is careful to reiterate that the motives toward fetal life need not and should not be any different from the motives toward maternal life. To want to save the mother does not entail as a necessary correlate to want to kill the fetus. All that the direct action against the fetus need comprehend is an intention to incapacitate the fetus and thereby prevent its threat to maternal (and in these cases of mutual mortal conflict, its own) life. Hence, "in this situation it is correct to say that the intention of this action is not the killing, not the death, of the fetus, but the incapacitation of it from carrying out the material aggression that it is effecting upon the life of the mother." Ramsey concludes from this approach that no moral evil is done in such an instance of direct abortion because the agent in his action neither wanted nor intended the death of another human being, but only the incapacitation of a life materially aggressing with fatal force upon another.[40]

In a more recent essay Ramsey takes account of the prospect in the immediate future for the "morning after" pill and argues that this medication can be morally justified as a "retroactive contraceptive" but not as an abortifacient. His distinction here is not altogether clear to me in the light of *present* pharmacological preparations, and this could be another case of "a rose by any other name." Ramsey's worry, however, might be that sophistication of the "morning after" pill will render it effective up to *several* mornings after; and when that occurs we will not be deal-

[39] *Ibid.*, p. 15.
[40] *Ibid.*, pp. 16, 18.

ing with a simple matter of retroactive contraception but destruction of nascent life at some early stage of its germination.[41]

It is for this reason that Ramsey addresses himself to a question which he earlier thought of little consequence; namely, *when* it is that germinating life can claim to be a fit subject of protection and be thereby accorded the sanctity and dignity of a human person. Of three possibilities—i.e., the time of implantation or nidation (normally in the second week following fertilization), the time of blastocyst (the name given to the cluster of cells when they arrive in the uterus, usually about a week after fertilization), and the moment of origin of the genotype (impregnation)—Ramsey opts for the stage of blastocyst and argues that this is the point at which the first origins of *individual* human life can be established.[42] In so doing, he has chosen a genetic account of the arrival of the essential constitutive features of a human individual, an account which, in his judgment, permits development of a moral argument adequate to justify attacking prehuman matter (i.e., before blastocyst). Moreover, he has defined rather precisely when direct destruction of nascent life may be undertaken (before blastocyst) and when that life is protected against all but indirect attack (after blastocyst), *except* for those situations in which *both* fetal and maternal life will be forfeited unless the fetus is fatally incapacitated.

Ramsey has introduced a stringent note (uncharacteristic of much Protestant reflection on abortion) into the discussion, and what he contends deserves careful consideration by every Christian who wants to take seriously the questions surrounding abortion in the context of modern medicine, genetics, and microbiology. Ramsey's reflections, however, have led him to a kind of "genetic determinism." In one sense it is certainly true that who one is and is ever going to be was determined at the moment of impregnation; but there is another, and I think more profoundly individual and personal, sense in which genetic and biological factors are better understood as *preconditional for* rather than as *definitive of* human life. The argument from blastocyst is not in

[41] Paul Ramsey, "Some Terms of Reference for the Abortion Debate," *Abortion*, ed. John T. Noonan (Cambridge: Harvard University Press, 1970).
[42] Cf. "The Sanctity of Life," p. 4, n. 1.

principle functionally different after all from the old animation arguments; what is different is that another arbitrary time has been assigned (i.e., before or after blastocyst) which can be argued in view of certain current data we have about the human reproductive process.

Moreover, we cannot fail to see the extended ways in which human and personal life, indeed genotypes themselves, are being historically shaped and conditioned in both intentional and unintentional ways. We are, for example, currently supplementing most of our stock cereal foods with vitamins to supply the requisite "daily minimum," prolonging life, eradicating disease and poverty, and declaring war on air and water pollution. But who is this man of the future that we are proceeding thus to build with such reckless abandon; and who has defined, in even a rudimentary way, what the biological, genetic, and other characteristics are that he should most desirably possess? That we are toying with the future in indiscriminate and sometimes unintentional ways is self-evident from any number of perspectives; and the practical bearing of this fact is simply that we are not allowing or depending upon purely natural attributes to shape life that is or is to be human. Indeed, why should we? There is no convincing reason that we should think of ourselves as the zenith (or, for that matter, the nadir) of the evolution of our species, unimprovable and irreformable; indeed, there is considerable evidence to the contrary!

We need, finally, to comment on Ramsey's employment of the direct-indirect distinction. He argues that "to abort the fetus may be the foreknown, anticipated and permitted result of surgical or other emergency action whose *primary thrust* is directed to the end of saving the mother's life." [43] As in the case of Roman Catholic defenses of this distinction, however, the question of personal responsibility is too neatly circumscribed. Ramsey, together with Catholic moralists in general, fails to appreciate how one can act in the face of unavoidable and irremediable conflict without seeking refuge for the action taken in a social or historical fiction that attributes responsibility to an accidental or fated cir-

---

[43] "The Morality of Abortion," p. 79.

cumstance. We can agree that the *primary thrust* of human action ought in every context to be reconciling and not alienating, therapeutic and not destructive, charitable and not malicious. But contending thus does not excuse those actions which, in the conflicting situations of competing neighbor love, *appear* to be unloving.

Values are virtually always competing in the decision-making arena—as, for example, in Nazi Germany, where the obligation to truth-telling was frequently in conflict with the obligation to preserve life. What is needed is not a simple reference to the inviolability of this or that, or even every, life because of its genetic constitution, nor a principle of expiation whereby real guilt and remorse are neatly camouflaged by sharp differentiations among mixed intentions. Surely there is a sense in which the death of the fetus is *not* desired or intended in the decisional process *antecedent* to abortion; and one struggles to find alternative procedures which, if feasible, will release him from an apparently irremediable conflict and offer the prospect of preserving *both* lives. But when it is established that the conflict is genuinely irremediable, the choices are narrowed to only two: namely, the choice to preserve the life of the one or the choice to preserve the life of the other. In either option, the choice made has *direct* consequences for both lives; and it might be said, however crudely but never callously, that the fetus' life was the price paid for the mother's life, or vice-versa!

To fail to acknowledge the full implication of such a decision is a denial of all the perceptions that occasioned and issued in the original decision. And it is of questionable service to the sensible conscience to suggest that responsibility for an act is mitigated by lack of intention to do it! The fact is that one does mean to do "it"—not, it may be granted, as the *primary* thrust but surely as a corollary of that primary thrust (that is, as an unavoidable and foreknown consequence in the train of that primary thrust and necessary to its achievement)—and meaning to do it, one does it. Now it would seem to me better in every respect frankly to acknowledge this and learn to live with it. The capacity to live in such tension is grounded in awareness of grace; i.e., the burden of having directly decided between two competing lives

46

would be intolerable if one did not appreciate that his own acceptance before God, like that of others, is unconditional.

No Protestant theologian in the twentieth century has argued more exhaustively or persuasively for the triumph of grace than Karl Barth; and an example of this is the general theological framework within which the question of the distinctly human is treated in the *Church Dogmatics* III/2. What allows us to speak of man as essentially human, what makes a man a man, is best expressed, said Barth, as an "ontological determination." By this term he meant that man's identity as man, together with his reason for being, is referable first and last to the fact that he is a being with God: Jesus has indwelt our history; we have been made God's covenant partner; we are both from and to God. In other words, man is essentially a *history*; but he is a special history that entails knowledge of God's grace, obedience to God, the invocation of God, and freedom in God. True and essential humanity, therefore, consists in relationship, and it is for this reason that Barth characterizes our possibility to be human in terms of *analogia relationis*.

Abortion and cognate issues are discussed in the *Church Dogmatics* III/4, and specifically in the context of elucidating the meaning of the commandment, "Thou shalt not kill." In his typically dialectical fashion, Barth argues that affirmation and negation are alternately embraced in decision-making. In the same breath that one says yes to one value or preference he must simultaneously modify (or even negate) that commitment by saying yes to another value; and that if it were not that we are obliged to decide some things *now*, this dialectic would or could go on indefinitely.

The following extended quotation from Barth himself describes the process:

Human life—one's own and that of others—belongs to God. It is His loan and blessing. . . . Therefore respect is due to it, and, with respect, protection against each and every callous negation and destruction. Obedient abstention from such destruction, and therefore the obedient protection of life, will naturally include knowledge of its limitation. It is not divine life, but creaturely. It is not the eternal life promised to man, but temporal. . . . Thus the protection of life required of us is not unlimited nor absolute. It is simply the protection which God wills to demand of man as the Creator of this life and the Giver of the future eternal life. . . . It simply refers to the fact that human life has no absolute greatness or supreme value, that it is not a kind of second god. . . . But since human life is of relative greatness and limited value, its protection may also consist *ultima ratione* in its surrender and sacrifice.[44]

Barth's treatment of abortion as a particular issue begins, perhaps as an effort to re-establish respect for nascent life, with an assessment of embryonic autonomy very like what we have already seen in Thielicke and Bonhoeffer. The embryo, says Barth, is autonomous because it possesses its own brain, neurological and circulatory systems. It is not merely a part of the maternal whole, and it is its relative independence that establishes nascent species life as a "human being in its own right." Thus it is that "he who destroys germinating life kills a man and thus ventures the monstrous thing of decreeing concerning the life and death of a fellowman whose life is given by God and therefore, like his own, belongs to Him." [45] From this perspective, one answers the question of abortion with a definite *no*.

But human life, including germinating life, is not an absolute or supreme value, and "cannot claim to be preserved in all circumstances, whether in relation to God or to other men." [46] And it is this awareness which raises the possibility of the exceptional case, that is, the situation in which the destruction of nascent life is not prohibited but positively enjoined. If there is indeed this possibility, there must also be the corresponding possibility of forgiveness for this action in the measure to which it "ventures the monstrous thing" of decreeing life and death to one whose life is given by, and belongs only to, God.

Because the command of God is based on his grace, Barth has no doubt that this possibility is sometimes actualized. There are situations in which, after all the arguments for inviolability are considered, abortion becomes the *ultima ratio*. These are certainly

[44] *Church Dogmatics* III/4, trans. A. T. Mackay, *et al.* (Edinburgh: T. & T. Clark, 1961), 397-98.

[45] *Ibid.*, p. 416.

[46] *Ibid.*, p. 420.

exceptional cases, including irremediable conflict between nascent and maternal lives in which both will die unless the fetus is destroyed but also extending to the choice between the life or health of the mother and that of the fetus. Even in these latter instances, in Barth's judgment, "the destruction of the child in the mother's womb might be permitted and commanded." [47]

Such a decision, even on these grounds, remains difficult and ambiguous, and Barth concludes his essay on abortion with several provisional guidelines which are offered as assistance in calculating the theological risks. But his main interest for us here is the unique way in which he has maintained a viable relationship, however taut, between two rather different views of what it is that constitutes *humanitas*. He has referred to human life—whether nascent or mature—in both naturalistic and relational categories, and offered a model for decision-making which allows both commandment and situation to assert their relative bearing in ways that are activated, rather than paralyzed, by finite ambiguity and uncertainty.

VI

There is a certain value in having reviewed these several reflections on the theological and moral issues posed by abortion; they remind us, if sometimes only obliquely and by implication, that a profoundly complex and intricate cluster of variables informs discriminating choice, when that choice has to be made, between nascent and mature human life. Careful analysis has further revealed that characteristic of these approaches is a certain presuppositional frame within which most of them work; and this is that human species life, at some more or less determinate point in its biological or genetic becoming, is (or ought to be) inviolable and sacrosanct. The popular corollary is that there is a little bit of God in each of us—a "spark of the divine," as it is sometimes described —and that any human tampering with this is not among the things over which man has been given dominion.

I have wanted to argue, however, that so long as we insist upon

[47] *Ibid.*, p. 421.

a substantive theory of "soul," in whatever sophisticated modern sense, we are obliged to reflect upon and treat our relation to it as the objectification of a category of meaning which is fundamentally relational in character. "Soul" is not a substance; rather, it is best understood as a word which signifies the lasting value-in-relationship which we attach and attribute to human beings. Moreover, that value is perceived and affirmed, as all values are, in relationship. There is no biblical notion of a disembodied soul; nor, for that matter, does the Bible support a body-soul dualism. Man, biblically understood, is both biological organism and responsible self—and this is an affirmation as congenial to modern thought as it is to the ancient wisdom of the Bible. Whatever else "soul" may mean in our commonsense use of the word, it is a relational and not a substantive category.

Christians have never appropriately located the sanctity of persons in metabolizing life *per se*. Authentic life, as Matthew 6:25 says, is more than food, and the body more than clothing. We might paraphrase to say that to be a human person entails more than having a body, that to be a human person is not merely a matter of statically being a certain kind of substance. Substance of some sort is certainly preconditional to becoming personal—in the same way that food is preconditional to life, and body to clothing —but what we mean by "personal" is transcendent of bare substance. Empirically a person is always in process, always becoming personal. In addition, John 10:10, citing Jesus' words, "I am come that they might have life, and that they might have it more abundantly," seems to presuppose that there is no life without relationship with God in Christ. Life, as Barth and others eloquently maintain, is a *gift* from God. But even this assertion may require "personal" qualification; at least it is fitting to question whether nascent life which results from rape or prostitution is gifted to us by God. We do not, after all, require a personalizing relationship with God in order to procreate in the biological sense.

The location of fetal immunity in the concept of substantial soul furthermore presumes to know that the initiating time of God's relationship with his creature has already occurred. Even granting that it is the *relationship* which is inviolable, and that "soul" is the symbol for the relationship, it nevertheless seems to me that a considerable measure of agnosticism is empirically wise regarding the initiating time of God's never-to-be-severed relationship. Given our human resources, to designate a specific time with respect to this relationship is both arbitrary and hubristic. It may be that, in a particular instance of abortion, God *has already initiated* his personalizing relationship; and if this be so, God may yet require (not as punishment but as a further service of love) some eschatological reconciliation. But this way of talking, even with supportive theological argumentation, is an implicate of other theological affirmations at best (or metaphysical speculation at worst!).

That the notion of an eternal and indestructible "soul" which is innate in the species is more akin to speculative Greek philosophy than to the New Testament gospel need not preoccupy us here. Indeed, even if the basic Greek notion were granted, we would still face the impressive question: When is "soul" present in human existence? Some theologians are agreed on the point that man is distinguished from the lower animals, at least in part, by the presence of "soul"; conversely, there is rather wide diversity among theological opinions, as we have seen, as to precisely *when* it is that God initiates his never-to-be-severed relationship with his creature. As regards this latter question, we cannot presume to date God's initiating personalization of any man, and therefore a considerable measure of agnosticism seems empirically wise.

The principal question of abortion thus remains to be adjudicated by human reason, compassion, fidelity, understanding, and all else that constitutes our creaturely apparatus for making morally sensitive and discriminating and finite judgments. That question is, simply, *when is life human?* The answer is neither simple nor arbitrary. It may be that, in some ultimate sense, the criteria for answering the question reside in either personal or biological categories; meantime, however, it seems still feasible to me that a comprehensive, holistic perspective most adequately incorporates the salient features of both. It is relatively easy, I know, to assert that the old bifurcations between man and nature, or subjective and objective, or history and nature, are mistaken and that our decisional dilemma is misplaced if we locate it between these (presumably) antagonistic polarities. But it is much more difficult to state with precision just how these apparent antitheses are related aspects of a single reality. That, nevertheless, is what is at stake here: an affirmation of the dignity of man which transcends but is not discontinuous with nature.

It is plain that we do not yet have a well-articulated consensus on what constitutes the category of "personal." But that predicament is understandable, and can even be celebrated, when we acknowledge that "personal" is always a category referable to becoming and process rather than being and fixity. On the other hand, neither do we all agree that biologism, of one or another sort, is an unambiguous and undifferentiated premise for defining *humanum*. William Temple once argued that reality is best conceived as a series of grades or strata, designated in ascending order as matter-life-mind-spirit, which are dialectically interrelated. The lower grades, he said, find their fullness of being and meaning only when used by the higher grades as instruments of self-expression; conversely, the higher grades require the lower ones for their actualization. In this way, each is necessary to the other in order to embody or symbolize what is more than itself alone.[48]

But personality is always transcendent in relation to process, and purpose differs from organic action and reaction; it therefore makes sense to contend that the decisively crucial desideratum in matters affecting *humanum* is personality or selfhood. On that assumption, I think it arguable that decisional emphasis vis-à-vis abortion deserves to be placed on the relational character of the context in which choice has to be made. That this is a provisional and tentative judgment in any case, and subject to change as experience and data alter perception, is presupposed. And to the argument that this way of doing ethics would do violence to *some* fetuses, I would only respond that operating from other premises (perhaps biological or genetic) also does violence to *some* fetuses —and if not in the womb, then certainly in the world of their becoming mature creatures. Indeed, if the premise be accepted that biological existence is preconditional to, but not definitive of, personalizing and personalized life, I believe it arguably the part

[48] William Temple, *Christus Veritas* (London: MacMillan & Co., 1964).

of mercy and reason to foreclose the birth of nascent life which is or promises to be severely deformed, defective, or disadvantaged.

In the last analysis, one must assume his *human* responsibility, with all that this entails—principally, the limitations of creatureliness. Man is not God, and remembrance of that alleviates the customary (and perhaps only human) ambition and pressure for fault-free and unambiguously good decision-making. In the present situation—i.e., without intending to speak for all times and situations—it is therefore reasonable, and even fitting, to suppose that different people will decide differently about similar moral issues. One couple may decide to terminate a pregnancy which holds a statistically negligible promise of viable human relationships, while another couple may not. The particular mix of any given decisional moment is impressively relevant in view of the fact that responsibility, in interpersonal relationships, is never unilateral and that consideration of more than a fetal life is, by definition, at stake in circumstances which call for such a choice to be made. A couple with *no* children and little or no prospect of another pregnancy might elect to risk carrying to term a fetus exposed in the first trimester to rubella; another couple, with other children and prospect for other pregnancies, if wanted, might choose to abort.

This is neither strange nor bizarre moral logic. We repudiate tyranny in all human relationships; fetal tyranny, merely because it is fetal, is no exception. Moreover, we cannot hide behind the facade of impersonal nature or a *Deus ex machina* as justification for indecision and inaction. Direct abortion, when it is unavoidable, is no more than honest confrontation with this fact of our creatureliness and the dilemma of limited alternatives. We might wish that the alternatives were different, or that our choice-options were larger; but wishing does not make it so.

Finally, it warrants saying that abortion is not murder; it is abortion, and no intelligent purpose is served by continuing to insist on the mutuality and correspondence of these two actions. Abortion is a particular moral issue with its own moral problematics. It involves mature people in a morally discriminating decision to terminate nascent life; it is a premeditated but not thereby malicious action; it can, and ought always to be, a genuinely regrettable alternative to unwanted pregnancy; and claim for fetal value, like the value for any life at whatever stage of its development, is inescapably relative to the cluster of other values which impinge upon the decision to abort or not to abort a given pregnancy.

II

The Meaning of Human Parenthood

It is not unusual for a procedure which was regarded in its formative stages as a medical curiosity to become a relatively safe and even recommended treatment for alleviation of some human debility or disease. Artificial insemination is such a procedure. Until comparatively recent times, childless couples were obliged either to accommodate themselves to a "barren marriage" or secure children through adoption or adultery (presuming in the latter instance that the wife is not sterile). Now, however, artificial insemination provides another alternative to childlessness. As a means by which sterility may be overcome and pregnancy stimulated, AI complements our capacity to restrain fecundity through conception control. With these capabilities we have the means, if not always the wisdom, for exercising intentional and purposive control over the generation of life, and—of special interest to us in this context—for controlling the generation of our own species life.

Artificial insemination is a much more recent capability than conception control. As we indicated earlier, abortifacient recipes have been known for over 4,500 years, and contraception, by one or another means, is a practice which doubtless antedates recorded history. Probably the earliest recorded discussion of artificial insemination occurs in a second-century A.D. Talmudic text, which hypothesizes the moral status of a woman who had been accidentally impregnated in bath water previously used by a man.[1] But this kind of fortuitous situation is not what we are concerned with here; besides being technically very problematic, it is accidental. Rather, we are interested in whether artificial insemination, which is now technically feasible in many instances of otherwise childless marriages, is morally licit as an intentional means of overcoming sterility and/or infecundity.

I

Artificial insemination is a procedure which consists of depositing semen, with the aid of instruments, in the vagina, cervical canal, or uterus with the intention of causing pregnancy which, by ordinary sexual union, is deemed unlikely or impossible. AI is basically of two types: homologous, when the semen is obtained from the husband (AIH); and heterologous, when the semen is secured from a donor (AID). Because spermatozoa may be separated from seminal plasma, however, it is possible to confuse or combine a husband's spermatozoa with a donor's seminal plasma (in order, for example, to increase sperm motility). In this circumstance, the process is properly called AIH inasmuch as the donor cannot be responsible for conception. On relatively rare occasions the husband's and donor's spermatozoa are combined in order to increase the possibilities for producing pregnancy while retaining the odd chance that the husband's sperm will be responsible for fertilization. This latter procedure is designated AIHD or CAI (combined artificial insemination), and ordinarily undertaken more for emotional than biological reasons.

The common conditions underlying the election of one or the other of these types of AI include impotency or sterility of the husband, genital debility or malformation in either spouse, dyspareunia (i.e., pain or difficulty in intercourse), genetic incompatibility (for example, Rhesus factors), or hereditary disease.

The history of experimentation with AI is itself relatively brief. Prior to the eighteenth century there are only a few isolated ref-

[1] Kardimon, "Artificial Insemination in the Talmud," *The Hebrew Medical Journal* (1942), 2:164.

erences to the practice. Arab horse-breeders were said to have impregnated brood mares by artificial means as early as the fourteenth century; Ludwig Jacobi successfully fertilized fish in 1742; and Lazario Spallanzani achieved fecundation in a spaniel bitch (which bore three puppies!) in 1780. The first successful artificial insemination in humans occurred in the late eighteenth century when John Hunter accomplished the feat with the wife of a London linen draper.[2] There followed other successful AIH experiments in France and the United States, and in 1909 an AID experiment, performed twenty-five years earlier, was reported by an American doctor.[3]

Meanwhile, Gregor Mendel had concluded his garden pea experiments which showed that in sexually reproduced organisms two factors are responsible for each single characteristic in offspring. These factors were later formulated as the chromosomal basis for controlling and predicting heredity. Now we know that in human cells there are twenty-three pairs of chromosomes which contain the genetic material DNA, and that in human reproduction sperm and ovum each contain exactly half the chromosomes originally present (i.e., twenty-three unpaired chromosomes) so that at fertilization a new set of twenty-three pairs occurs. These two processes—the techniques of artificial insemination and the discovery of the genetic bases of heredity—have only recently been seriously related, and together they give rise to a number of far-reaching questions. In the early twentieth century AI was largely restricted to experiments in animal husbandry and horticulture, and it is only within recent years that clinics have been established to provide medically supervised AI as an alternative to involuntary childlessness. Because of the secrecy which, for many reasons, surrounds this operation, it is difficult to obtain precise statistics regarding the number of attempts made or live births obtained from AI, both homologous and heterologous. It is estimated, however, that up to 150,000 living Americans owe their births to

[2] Philosophical Transactions of the Royal Society of London (1799), 18:162; cited in Norman St. John-Stevas, *Life, Death and the Law*, p. 117.
[3] A. D. Hard, "Artificial Impregnation," *The Medical World* (1909), 27:163 ff.

AI,[4] and that AI pregnancies are currently being achieved at the rate of about 10,000 per year.[5]

II

Legal interest in artificial insemination is almost entirely restricted to AID, and lawyers generally agree that AIH creates only minor problems in the event that there is subsequent effort to dissolve the marriage by divorce or nullity on grounds of non-consummation. An English court has held that AIH, in a case in which the husband was psychologically incapable of intercourse but the wife had been artificially impregnated with her husband's semen, neither ratifies the marriage nor bars a nullity decree. More specifically, the court decided that the wife's submission to AIH did not constitute acceptance on her part of her husband's impotency, and thus surrender of her marital rights.[6] Happily there are also statutes in most jurisdictions which, in the event of a ruling such as this, prevent the child of the "marriage" from being bastardized at the time the decree is issued.

This appears to be another instance of the law's real difficulty, if not inability, to apply ancient principles to certain modern problems. At least it would seem no longer useful, in fact it is inaccurate in cases of AIH, to revert to precedents pertaining to sterility and impotence as grounds for divorce or nullity. But more important than the distinction between sterility and impotency, which doubtless needs more careful legal attention, there are larger questions which bear upon the authenticity of marriage which can no longer be—and never were appropriately—considered in terms of biological mechanics alone.

The legal problems occasioned by AID are more serious and chiefly of two sorts: (1) the status of children conceived by AID

[4] "The Riddle of A.I." *Time,* February 25, 1966, p. 48.

[5] Arthur C. Christakos, "Human Genetic Manipulation: Fact and Fancy," *Duke Alumni Register* (1968), 54:2.

[6] George C. Christie, "Some Thoughts on the Legal Problems Raised by the Prospect of Genetic Manipulation," *Duke Alumni Register* (1968), 54:5. Cf. Glanville Williams, *The Sanctity of Life and the Criminal Law* (New York: Alfred A. Knopf, 1957), pp. 118 ff.; and St. John-Stevas, *Life, Death and the Law,* p. 121.

and the rights and responsibilities of the husband of an artificially impregnated wife; and (2) whether AID constitutes adultery and thus grounds for divorce. The American press has recently reported two court actions which address, even if they do not resolve, these issues.

The status of children and the responsibility of husbands were at issue in Sonoma County, California, in the March, 1967, trial of F. J. Sorensen. Because of Mr. Sorensen's sterility, both he and Mrs. Sorensen had consented to AID as a remedy for their childless marriage. Subsequently Mrs. Sorensen was artificially inseminated, became pregnant, and gave birth to Christopher in 1961. Three years later Mr. and Mrs. Sorensen were divorced, but Mrs. Sorensen refused at that time to accept any financial support from her husband. In 1966, when Mrs. Sorensen became ill and applied for welfare support, the district attorney charged her husband with violation of a state statute which makes willful nonsupport of a legitimate child a misdemeanor. Municipal Court Judge James E. Jones, Jr., ruled that Mr. Sorensen was guilty as charged on the principle that "all children born in wedlock are presumed the legitimate issue of the marital partners." [7]

A number of factors, however, make Judge Jones's decision somewhat less than definitive; and these relate not so much to the legal obligations of parents for children as to the legal formulation of parenthood itself. Most lawyers would probably agree with Judge Jones's conclusion that conception from a donor's semen is no bar to legitimacy when birth occurs within wedlock and with the husband's consent.[8] In the Sorensen case, however, the presumption of legitimacy could perhaps have been rebutted by evidence that Mr. Sorensen's sterility clearly precluded his being Christopher's father. In that event, and unless Judge Jones was prepared to argue that Mr. Sorensen had adopted Christopher *de facto* in consenting to the AID which produced his conception, there would have been little *legal* alternative to declaring the child a bastard and relieving the husband of any responsibility in respect to him. Currently only one state (Oklahoma, since May,

[7] "The Child of Artificial Insemination: Status and Rights," *Time*, April 14, 1967, pp. 79-80.
[8] Williams, *The Sanctity of Life*, p. 118.

1967) legislatively recognizes the legitimacy of AI children; [9] there is no federal statute affecting this question, and judicial precedent is far from being well established.[10] Thus, beyond establishing Mr. Sorensen's culpability in the matter at issue, there are the additional questions of donor liability and the AI child's inheritance rights. If evidence of Mr. Sorensen's sterility had rebutted the presumption of Christopher's legitimacy, would this have meant that the donor might be liable for child support under the bastardy statutes? [11] And since inheritance ordinarily depends upon legitimacy, would rebuttal of the presumption of Christopher's legitimacy deny him all rights in respect of his mother's husband?

These are delicate and complex issues which can no longer be resolved by uncomplicated reference to biological cause and effect. AI makes it technically feasible now for a single individual to sire hundreds or thousands of offspring, at the rate of approximately thirty pregnancies per donation; and while individual contribution to reproduction in such magnitude is highly unlikely, it is nevertheless statistically possible. Much more probable is a situation in which the same donor may impregnate several different wives, especially since it is no longer necessary to use "fresh" semen. A biologist at the University of Michigan's Center for Research in Reproductive Biology recently reported that twenty-nine women had been made pregnant by male sperm *frozen* for up to two and one half years! [12] The tragic figure in these situations is, of course, the child produced by AID; and it is for his sake preeminently that these questions deserve prompt, compassionate, and comprehensive attention.

The other major legal issue raised by AID is whether this op-

[9] Oklahoma Stat. Ann. tit. 10, 551, 552 (Supp. 1967).

[10] The New York Supreme Court, in 1948, in Strnad v. Strnad, held an artificially inseminated child to be legitimate and therefore granted Mr. Strnad visitation rights after separation. Mrs. Strnad, however, moved to Oklahoma and in litigation there the New York decision was nullified and Mrs. Strnad given exclusive custody. Other cases on record tend to rule in favor of illegitimacy of AID offspring, even in those instances where the husband gave his consent.

[11] An Arizona statute (Arizona Code 1939, ch. 27:401) provides that "every child is the legitimate child of its natural parents." Cf. Williams, *The Sanctity of Life*, p. 121.

[12] Associated Press Dispatch, April 7, 1966.

eration is technically an instance of adultery. The underlying assumption which gives this question force is the notion that marriage is fundamentally constituted by exclusive bodily rights to the reproductive capacities of husband and wife. In 1966 a Manhattan internist, John M. Prutting, sued his wife for divorce on the grounds of adultery. Without his consent or knowledge, claimed the doctor, his wife had conceived a child by AID.[13]

Judicial opinions (more often *dicta* than rulings) have varied, but it is probably fair to say that their greater weight has tended in favor of the view that AID *without consent by both spouses* violates the marriage contract. In the 1921 Canadian case of Orford v. Orford, Judge Orde denied a plea for alimony in a case involving an AID child which was conceived without the husband's consent. For the limited purpose of determining responsibility for maintenance, Judge Orde held that "the criterion of adultery is not sexual intercourse (as the common law holds) but the voluntary surrender by a wife of her reproductive faculties to another person." [14] The logical application of this opinion, however, would require naming the donor as co-respondent in the action; and if the donor were married, this could in turn involve the recipient wife as co-respondent in divorce action brought by the donor's wife! But this begins to strain common sense. In 1945, in the Cook County (Illinois) Circuit Court, Judge Feinberg ruled that AID does not constitute "grounds for divorce on a charge of adultery," because the donor's act is too remote from the actual insemination to establish his complicity.[15] Judge Feinberg might have extended his logic to argue that if the wife's reproductive faculties were in fact surrendered to another person, that person would arguably be the doctor who performed the operation and not the donor who, as it were, merely contributed the "raw material" but had nothing to do with its eventual disposition or the particular genetic shape it might take as a "finished product"; but this line of reasoning would be simply erroneous.

[13] *Time*, February 25, 1966, p. 48.
[14] Cited in Fletcher, *Morals and Medicine*, p. 108. Cf. Williams, *The Sanctity of Life*, p. 123; and St. John-Stevas, *Life, Death and the Law*, p. 130.
[15] Fletcher, *Morals and Medicine*, pp. 108-9. Cf. Williams, *The Sanctity of Life*, p. 124.

Judge Orde had stated for the Supreme Court of Ontario that "If it was necessary to do so, I would hold that [AID] in itself was 'sexual intercourse.' " [16] This statement doubtless helps to dramatize the problem of defining adultery more precisely for legal purposes; I am told that most United States lawyers would now tend to interpret adultery as sexual intercourse which involves carnal contact. If this is in fact the situation, it appears unlikely that AID without consent might constitute legal grounds for divorce by reason of adultery. AID without consent does, however, undoubtedly violate the marriage covenant in ways that deserve careful and discriminating articulation. And although such an operation may not be adultery in a proper and inclusive sense, it is comparable to the semantic distinction sometimes conferred upon the "technical virgin," who may engage in heavy petting to the point of mutual masturbation but draws the line at what is conventionally signified by coition. In both AID and mutual masturbation the venereal and procreative aspects of human sexuality have been neatly sundered.

In view of relatively recent developments in molecular biology and biomedicine, the most urgent ethical questions which emerge from our capacity to engineer AI and genetic manipulation have bearing, I think, upon (1) the implications of artificial impregnation for our understanding of marriage and other personal dimensions of relationship, such as parenthood, and (2) the limits and obligations which are appropriate for human control over human life in light of the increasing capacity for determining our genetic future.

III

It has long been held by Christians that marriage is the human context for reproduction and that, indeed, procreation and its attendant parental responsibility is a primary purpose of marriage. The passage in Genesis 1:28, "be fruitful and multiply," has frequently been taken to be definitive of the purpose and obligation of marriage; although, at least since Augustine, marriage has

---

[16] Cited in Williams, *The Sanctity of Life*, p. 125.

also been tolerated by Christians as a concession to concupiscence and an apparently irrepressible sexual lust.

As recently as 1968, Pope Paul VI, in his encyclical *Humanae Vitae*, reaffirmed that for Roman Catholics the regulative principle of human sexual congress is "the transmission of life"—and thus forbade again the employment by Catholics of direct and "artificial" interventions for the control of conception. But procreation is not, as is sometimes mistakenly thought, the *only* end of marriage; the fostering of mutual love, together with the allaying of concupiscence, are acknowledged by Catholic moralists as secondary or subordinate ends.[17] Nevertheless, priorities are important, as Pope Pius XII indicated in an address to Italian midwives:

The use of the natural inclination to generate is lawful only in matrimony, in the service of and according to the order of the ends of marriage. . . . If nature had aimed exclusively or even primarily at a mutual gift and mutual possession of couples for pleasure . . . then the Creator would have adopted another plan in the formation and constitution of the natural act. But this act is completely subordinated to and ordered in accordance with the sole great law of *"generatio et educatio prolis,"* the fulfilling of the primary end of matrimony as the origin and source of life.[18]

On the surface this is a straightforward and uncomplicated position; but the assumptions, both implied and explicit, which

[17] The Pastoral Constitution on the Church in the Modern World, one of the documents of the Second Vatican Council, does indeed support mutual love as an essential end of marriage: "Marriage to be sure is not instituted solely for procreation. Rather, its very nature as an unbreakable compact between persons, and the welfare of the children, both demand that the mutual love of the spouses, too, be embodied in a rightly ordered manner, that it grow and ripen. Therefore, marriage persists as a whole manner and communion of life, and maintains its value and indissolubility, even when offspring are lacking." (Walter M. Abbott, ed., *The Documents of Vatican II* [New York: Guild Press, Association Press, and American Press, 1966], p. 255). The official status of this document deserves attention, especially within the context of this discussion, and an explanatory note is appended to its title: it is "a document that of its nature does not define or decree immutable dogma." (*Ibid.*, p. 199.)

[18] Pius XII, "Address to the Italian Catholic Union of Midwives," *Moral Questions Affecting Married Life* (Washington: National Catholic Welfare Conference, 1952), pp. 21-22.

inform this view have very far-reaching implications for the whole range of human actions which relate to sexual relationships. In sum, the classical Catholic position claims to derive the purpose of coition from the "very nature of the sex act itself." It holds, moreover, that pleasure, mutuality, and the unitive ends of intercourse are *in principle* secondary and subordinate to the primary and principal end of procreation and its corresponding responsibility for care and education of offspring.

In consequence of this approach, the morality of human sexual intercourse for Catholics is officially determined by its conformity to these antecedently specified rubrics. (I say "officially determined" because I am told by Catholic moralists that most Catholics today reject the primary-secondary formulation, as well as the underlying theory on which the formulation is based.) Coition must occur only between husband and wife; it must also be an act designed for procreation and unimpeded, by direct means, from achieving that goal. Specifically, human sexual congress, in order to be authentic, must involve intravaginal ejaculation by the husband and retention of the semen (or at least no deliberate effort at expulsion) by the wife.[19] It is for this reason that impotency constitutes an impediment to marriage and, if undiscovered prior to establishing marriage, adequate ground for nullity in both canon and civil law.[20] Sterility, however, is no impediment to marriage; nor is it, whether in the husband or the wife, sufficient ground for annulment of marriage! Consistency of argument would seem to require that *any* impediment to genuine intercourse would constitute suitable grounds for dissolution and nullity. The Catholic position is not thus reasoned, however, and I therefore simply report it.

[19] Cf. John P. Kenny, *Principles of Medical Ethics* (Cork, Ireland: Mercier Press, 1953), pp. 68-69. Fr. Kenny leaves no doubt that this is an unequivocal moral requirement: "In itself, per se, it [i.e., marital intercourse] must be an action from which generation can follow, even though, accidentally, it may happen that conception is impossible, either because of pregnancy or because of sterility. . . . The question as to whether or not conception is possible does not enter into the moral consideration."

[20] Canon 1068 declares: "Impotency anterior to the marriage and perpetual, whether in the man or in the woman, whether known to the other party or not, whether absolute or relative, annuls marriage by the very law of nature."

One further comment on the nature of marriage, from the Catholic perspective, is in order; and this is that marriage entails exclusive bodily possession of each spouse by the other. The practical effect of understanding marriage as a physical monopoly relates to both adultery and artificial insemination and, somewhat less directly, to parenthood. Judge Orde's criterion for adultery as "the voluntary surrender by a wife of her reproductive faculties to another person" was doubtless formulated on this or a similar assumption, as was his willingness to "hold that [AID] in itself was 'sexual intercourse.' "

Whether AID constitutes adultery would appear to be a question first of all referable to one's understanding of marriage, and embracing the mystery of love and human sexuality as well as the consensual obligations of couples to each other, their offspring, and the larger community. Official Catholic teaching, however, locates the primary purpose of marriage in the generation and education of children, together with a particular understanding of what kind of action constitutes a licit conception. Because artificial impregnation, whether homologous or heterologous, substitutes another action for "natural sexual intercourse," it is held to be morally objectionable. Moreover, on the principle of exclusive bodily rights to sexual and reproductive organs by the married couple, AID is judged to be adulterous as the invasion of the wife's reproductive system by another not her husband. Finally, it deserves notice that AI is condemned because the act of insemination is not a personal act of love-union between the spouses. On these grounds Catholic doctrine rejects AI as immoral and unlawful.

These understandings of the nature and function of authentic marriage and coition have definite implications, of course, for the second of our major concerns; namely, the question of the limits and obligations appropriate for human control over our genetic destiny. We will return to this issue later, but the moral logic of the Catholic position can be briefly indicated now: (1) the requirement of intravaginal ejaculation by the husband and retention of the semen by the wife renders AI illicit as an unnatural, and hence unlawful, act; (2) marriage as a physical monopoly judges AID to be adulterous; (3) the limits of human control over human destiny are imposed by a certain understanding of "nature" together with a principle of noninterference in what is thus supposed to be "natural" processes.[21]

Official Catholic teaching about the nature and purpose of marriage and coition has tended, in sum, to naturalistic reductionism and doctrinaire insistence upon the inordinate importance of reproduction. Popular Protestantism, on the other hand, has tended to subjective sentimentality and exaltation of venereal pleasure at the expense of a comprehensive sexual responsibility; and advocates of both the old and new moralities have contributed, though in rather different ways, to this malaise.

IV

Proponents of conservative Protestant Christianity maintain that some acts, because they are specifically commanded in the Bible, are *ubique, semper et ab omnibus* the Christian obligation. Correspondingly, there are other acts which are everywhere, al-

[21] Objection to AI, even though the husband's sperm be employed, is typically grounded in (1) the requirement of retention by the wife of the husband's semen and (2) the prohibition against masturbation or any other form of what is mistakenly called "onanism." The first of these is clear enough, given the context of the argument. The Catholic interpretation of onanism, however, is considerably more problematic. Gen. 38:9 describes Onan's refusal to obey the law of levirate marriage and impregnate the wife of his deceased and childless brother. Official Catholic interpretation of this incident teaches that Onan's sin consisted in the "unnaturalness" of his act, i.e., extravaginal ejaculation. But this quite ignores the context and the explicit command which Onan disobeyed. Onan's sin was not against "natural intercourse" but against the Lord's command that he should perpetuate his dead brother's identity in Israel by providing progeny through the widow. (Cf. H. Wheeler Robinson, "The Hebrew Conception of Corporate Personality," *Beihefte zur Zeitschrift für die alttestamentliche Wissenschaft,* 66 [1936], 49-61.) In order to obtain semen, for either laboratory examination or AIH, some Catholic moralists have argued that semen procured (a) by aspiration from the epididymus or testicles, (b) by aspiration from the vagina *post coitam,* or (c) by cervical spoon or perforated condom is "probably lawful." These proposals remain unsettled, however; and meanwhile Pius XII's pronouncement condemning all forms of impregnation which do not involve "natural intercourse" suggests that these views may not be officially held. (Cf. Pius XII, "Address to the Italian Catholic Union of Midwives," pp. 19-20; and Pius XII, "Papal Address to the Fourth International Congress of Catholic Doctors," *Irish Ecclesiastical Record* [1950], 73:271-72.)

ways, and for everybody wrong because they are specifically forbidden by the Bible. It is this approach to truth and responsibility that has given warrant for the epithet that the Bible is the Protestant's "paper pope"; for, on these terms, the abiding element in God's revelation is located in the content of a particular command in the Bible which is eternally valid and unchanged, despite the participation of it and us in the relativity and flux of history.

Conservative Protestantism thus teaches that marriage and coition take their cue from the Bible and maintains that monogamous marriage is the biblical expression of God's unalterable and unambiguous will. Georgia Harkness, for example contends that the sciences of sociology and psychology only confirm what the Christian already knows as the divine will: "From both standpoints, monogamy is the only right form of marital relation." [22] And Carl F. H. Henry interprets the creation narratives, together with the Decalogue and the teachings of Jesus, as enforcing monogamous marriage: "The creation of a single male and from his side a female companion as his helpmeet, is to provide a permanent spiritual and moral basis for monogamous marriage." [23] Given this approach to the Bible, and the view of revelation which informs it, there is no ambiguity or equivocation about the appropriate context for human coition: one should either marry or abstain from sexual intercourse.

Probably owing to a preoccupation with correct behavior, together with the relative novelty of the issues we are specifically considering, there is no explicit instruction in the literature of conservative Protestantism on questions of artificial insemination and genetic manipulation. One might infer that AID would be morally objectionable as an invasion of monogamous monopoly, or that genetic engineering would qualify technically as an offensive sexual relation; but these judgments, however accurate, remain only inferences. What can be said in criticism of the so-called "old morality," and with specific reference to its own

[22] Georgia Harkness, *Christian Ethics* (Nashville: Abingdon Press, 1957), p. 129.
[23] Carl F. H. Henry, *Christian Personal Ethics* (Grand Rapids: Eerdmans Publishing Co., 1957), p. 273.

67

claims, is (1) that the Bible nowhere prescribes monogamy or prohibits polygamy, but simply commends marriage as a normal adult relationship;[24] (2) that the location of God's will in some given command of fixed content makes God's living presence superfluous and gives eloquent testimony to a Christianity *post mortem Dei*; and (3) that legalistic ethics deteriorates and moral sensitivity is blunted when rules become more important than persons and when institutions are taken as definitive of relationships.[25]

At the other end of the Protestant theological spectrum are those who argue that none of the biblical commandments, in their specific content, can be taken as the unambiguous and transparently clear expression of God's will. There are therefore no specified modes of conduct which are universally required of Christians. As Bishop John Robinson puts it, Jesus asks only that his disciples be open in every situation to the unconditional and absolute demand of love, "to subject everything in their lives to the overriding, unconditional claim of God's utterly gracious yet utterly demanding rule of righteous love." [26] Freed from bondage

[24] Cf. William Graham Cole, *Sex and Love in the Bible* (New York: Association Press, 1960), which is the most comprehensive statement of biblical views on sex and love yet published by a Protestant scholar. It also deserves noting in this context that modern biblical scholarship does not lend support to the exaltation of celibacy over marriage, a notion erroneously adopted by the Council of Trent in 1563 and reaffirmed as recently as 1954 by Pius XII in his encyclical *Sacra Virginitas* (*Acta Apostolicae Sedis*, [1954], 46:161-92).

[25] One of the obvious questions which arise from the moral insensitivity of legalistic ethics has to do with whether the spirit of adultery or lust may sometimes find expression *within marriage*; or with whether the institution of marriage, as a merely formal arrangement, adequately accounts for the possibility of a violation like rape *within marriage!* The error of legalism, in these and similar instances, lies in an objectification of language and behavior in which words like "marriage" and "rape" signify less a certain relationship (or lack of it) between persons than they do conformity with some antecedently prescribed and objective form of action.

[26] John A. T. Robinson, *Christian Morals Today* (Philadelphia: The Westminster Press, 1964), p. 12. A parallel statement occurs in Robinson's more widely read *Honest to God* (The Westminster Press, 1963), p. 114: "Life in Christ Jesus, in the new being, in the Spirit, means having no absolutes but his love, being totally uncommitted in every other respect but totally committed in this."

to prescriptions and codes and laws, the Christian is offered a direction, a cast, or style of life which liberates him for expressing *agape* in whatever circumstance. Amid the ambiguities and relativities of historical situations, what is "good" or "right" cannot be precisely anticipated and specified. New occasions do teach new duties.

No institution, then, can define relationships between persons; and sexual intercourse, according to Robinson, merely because it occurs within marriage, may be either right or wrong depending on the situation. It is not the marriage line that is decisive, but whether love is present or absent. When coition is honest and truthfully expresses the personal commitment ordinarily signified by this action, and when it serves but does not exploit the other person, it is presumably authentic whether or not a legal (or other institutionally validated) marriage has preceded this action.[27]

Liberal Protestant reflection on these questions appeals to both reason and conscience in its insistence that love is the only unconditional claim placed upon us, that the divine intention can never be located in the content of a particular command, and that nothing less than freedom from ethical rigorism and knowledge of situational problematics equip us for genuinely responsible decisions and actions.[28] Nevertheless, proponents of this view are liable to the basic criticisms made of all formal methods in ethics: (1) the essentially corporate character of the Christian life is not adequately recognized in exaggerated emphasis on individual responsibility; (2) failure to describe or define categories and concepts more precisely tends, in practice, to moral anarchy; and (3) unprincipled abandonment of law locates authority in the self alone and tends toward capriciousness in decision-making.

Despite the alternative which liberal Protestantism offers to the legalisms which derive from notions of both biblical and papal

---

[27] Cf. the similar qualification in Joseph Fletcher, *Situation Ethics: The New Morality* (Philadelphia: The Westminster Press, 1966), p. 140: "If people do not believe it is wrong to have sex relations outside marriage, it isn't, unless they hurt themselves, their partners, or others."

[28] Cf. Emil Brunner, *The Divine Imperative*, trans. Olive Wyon (Philadelphia: The Westminster Press, 1947), p. 134: "God's Command does not vary in *intention*, but it varies in *content*, according to the conditions with which it deals."

infallibility, the attempt to formulate responsible choices in biology and genetics in the present situation requires, simultaneously, more precise direction than is afforded by a vague admonition to show love, on the one hand, and less rigorous determination than is demanded by a naturalistic reductionism, on the other.

The Protestant theologian Helmut Thielicke has argued that AIH, to which both husband and wife mutually consent, does not transgress upon the essential and exclusive psychophysical relationship between them. No third person jeopardizes or invades the couple's one-flesh unity, and through the entire process they demonstrate their fidelity to each other. Moreover, even though masturbation may be involved,[29] this act cannot be extracted from the context which places it within a genuine bisexual fellowship and perceives it as instrumental to the fulfillment of this relationship. Thielicke thus argues that AIH in no way depersonalizes the intimate relationship between husband and wife, but in fact enhances it through loving fulfillment in procreation. There are, therefore, no serious reasons to object to homologous insemination on theological grounds.[30]

Artificial impregnation by donor is quite another matter, however, and Thielicke rejects this operation *in toto*. Not only is masturbation or other methods of securing donor semen separated from the marital I-Thou relationship but, more important, the psychophysical totality of the marriage is jeopardized by the introduction of a personal entity, the AID child, which incarnates the "existential fact" that the one-flesh unity between husband and wife is now divided. Thielicke's anxiety is not prompted by certainty that AID either is or will lead to infidelity, in the strict sense of that word, between spouses—though this, as a factor in the situation, is not ruled out; his apprehension is rather grounded in what he perceives to be certain unwarranted risks. He acknowledges concern that the biological father will be "deindividualized"

---

[29] There are several methods for obtaining semen, of which masturbation is only one. Alternative means include aspiration by puncture of the epididymus or testicles, post-coital aspiration from the vagina, post-coital use of a cervical spoon or tassette, rectal message of the prostate gland and seminal vesicles, condomistic intercourse, and coitus interruptus.

[30] *The Ethics of Sex*, pp. 252-58.

and "depersonalized" and thus rendered a nonperson in what is otherwise a profoundly personal experience; but Thielicke's real fear is that the AID child itself will have an extreme effect upon the marriage by signifying achievement of motherhood for the wife and failure of fatherhood for the husband. If this fear materialized, the indivisible psychophysical totality of the marriage would be ruptured; and that for Thielicke is a far worse abrogation of the marital covenant than involuntary childlessness. In the end, he advises that couples who are involuntarily childless must accept this deprivation as, in some sense, God's will for them and "suffer ethically" until a method can be developed which does not contradict the meaning of the sufferer's life.[31]

Thielicke rejects the notion that the absence of "natural sexual intercourse" is a moral impediment to conception. He shares with Catholic moralists, however, the view that marriage conveys—and is, in some sense, constituted by—exclusive bodily rights to sexual and reproductive organs, and that this is consistent with the notion that marriage between persons is fundamentally signified by a loving and unitive relationship. Had he developed substantial reasons for maintaining the principle of marital monopoly, his argument would have been more convincing; but merely hypothesizing several negative possibilities betrays what may be a more emotional and biological than rational and theological objection to AID. Moreover, Thielicke's most prominent hypothetical possibilities are grounded in naturalistic rather than personalitsic assumptions.

On the other hand, his claim that AID threatens marriage because it fulfills motherhood at the expense of confirming paternal failure shows great sensitivity for what parenthood in a non-biological sense may mean, and the general good success of adoption is significant support for Thielicke's point. Reciprocal mutual complementarity in interpersonal relations, especially in intimate relations like those of marriage and parenthood, is generally to be preferred to radical asymmetry; and thus the general preferability of adoption to AID. There are hundreds of thousands of adoptive parents who can lay no genetic or biologic claim to their

[31] *Ibid.*, pp. 258-68.

children but whose parenthood in relation to those children is indubitable; because parenthood is not defined by simple—or even complex!—fecundity, and to be a mother or a father or a child signifies more than mere breeding.

Joseph Fletcher has argued for a considerably more permissive attitude toward AI. Like Thielicke, he sees no serious objection to AIH as a means for overcoming childlessness; neither does he regard any of the noncopulative methods for obtaining the husband's semen for AIH as morally objectionable. Unlike Thielicke, however, Fletcher maintains that AID is compatible with a Christian understanding of sexuality, marriage, and parenthood. He regards any immediate threat of "stud breeding" of human beings as highly speculative and improbable, and dismisses the objection that AID involves sexual self-abuse (donor masturbation) on the grounds that masturbation loses its character as self-abuse "when it becomes the method or means to a procreative purpose which is otherwise impossible." [32] The most formidable objections to AID, according to Fletcher, lie in questions relating to marriage and parenthood; namely, whether AID constitutes adultery and whether the offspring thus produced are illegitimate. Fletcher answers no to both questions.

It is Fletcher's opinion that the marriage bond is not violated in AID because (1) marriage is not a physical monopoly, and mutual consent by husband and wife ensures that there is no broken faith between them, and (2) the wife's relationship with the donor is entirely impersonal.[33] Two claims, one of which is developed and the other of which is simply asserted, are advanced in support of this view.

Arguing against the notion that marriage is a physical monopoly, Fletcher maintains that polygamy, concubinage, and levirate marriage function in the Old Testament as prescientific AID surrogates.[34] Thus, he shows that Leah and Rachel sent their husband Jacob to conceive children by their handmaids (Gen. 30), that sterile Sarah sent her husband Abraham to her fecund maid Hagar (Gen. 16), and that Onan was commanded

[32] *Morals and Medicine*, p. 118.
[33] *Ibid.*, p. 121.
[34] *Ibid.*, pp. 119-21.

by his father to fulfill the levirate law by impregnating Tamar, the wife of Onan's dead and childless brother Er (Gen. 39). But this is a curious and exegetically dubious use of the Bible. Not only are the marital mores of the Old Testament far removed from the twentieth century, but in each of the instances cited the action precipitated equivocal if not negative consequences. Leah and Rachel suffered only temporary sterility, and both of them later bore children; indeed, Leah gave Jacob two sons and Rachel became the mother of Joseph (Gen. 30:17-24). Sarah was so offended by her pregnant maid's air of superiority that she banished both Hagar and her son Ishmael to the desert (Gen. 16:4-7); and later, when both she and Abraham were supposed to be well beyond their fertile years, Sarah gave birth to Isaac (Gen. 21:1-3). And Onan, as is generally well known, refused to impregnate Tamar, in consequence of which the Lord required his life (Gen. 38:9-10). Fletcher's use of the Old Testament to contradict monogamous monopoly is contrived and irrelevant to the present situation.

The second claim, that the personal character of the marital bond is not infringed by the impersonality of donor insemination, is simply asserted: "Artificial insemination mutually agreed upon by husband and wife does not involve any broken faith between them. . . . No personal relationship is entered into with the donor at all." [35] This seems fair enough on the face of it; but one questions whether it is really that simple and straightforward. Fletcher is doubtless right in his insistence that fidelity in marriage is "a *personal* bond between husband and wife, not primarily a legal contract" and that parenthood is "a *moral* relationship with children, not a material or merely physical relationship." [36] But he neglects to elaborate either the particular way in which he intends these statements or the freedom and obligation appropriate to such relationships. That there are certain assumed but unarticulated limits is apparent when one considers that AID in the case of a fertile husband but sterile wife is not even mentioned.

If it is so self-evident that AID is no invasion of marital chas-

[35] *Ibid.*, p. 121.
[36] *Ibid.*, p. 139.

tity owing to consent, impersonality of procedure, and all the rest, one might reasonably ask why no one, not even Fletcher, has seriously advocated anonymous egg and womb donors who would (for a fee, of course) receive a husband's sperm, be hostess to this nascent life until delivery, and thereby provide the same *technical* service as the sperm donor. It is arguable, of course, that sperm, or even egg, donation is markedly different from experiencing pregnancy, and that we are at least in another ball park, if not another ball game, when we discuss AID in this context. And so we are; because whatever the meaning we finally attach to words like "personal" and "human," it cannot be entirely separated from natural, physical, bodily processes. Fletcher's emphasis on the personal and relational is a needed corrective to the excessive legalism and objectivism that has for so long dehumanized the ethics of sex and marriage; but in his exuberance he has also made claims too extravagant to be supported by the facts.

If AID is to be convincingly recommended, other reasons for its justification must be put forward. Meantime, the arguments ordinarily advanced (that it provides an acceptable alternative to childlessness in cases of a husband's sterility, that it allows a couple to have a baby "at least half ours," and that it gives a wife the satisfactions of maternity) are inadequate; and the AID baby's procreation tends to signify more than it intends. Why this is so, however, requires careful examination of a Christian understanding of coition and procreation.

V

As the biologic occasion which makes possible the meeting of sperm and egg, human coition is *in principle* bound up with procreation—and, in our society, with marriage and family life. It deserves more careful notice than it often receives that the offspring of such a union is, as we conventionally say, procreated. But the use of the prefix *pro* is no semantic accident, and in the Judeo-Christian tradition we use it to signify and guard the fact that when human beings create, they do so on another's behalf— specifically, on God's behalf. Similarly, with the prefix *re*, as in reproduction, we point backward to an originating event which we recapitulate in our own time and place. In an important and profound sense, fecundation, pregnancy, and parturition are always a reoccurrence and we are not, in any precise sense, the creators *de novo* of our children. Navels are a constant reminder of that fact.

On the other hand, there is the obvious fact that children would not be conceived and born unless persons played their part; so it is probably more accurate, in the end, to say that we are immediately but not exclusively the parents of our children. Putting it that way suggests that there are many sorts of considerations—among them genetic, sociological, and theological—that hedge how we think about human sexuality and parenthood. To act on behalf of God is one of the impressive notions that derives from a theistic approach to human sexuality; and to procreate, to reproduce in any authentic sense, is thus to be aware that coitus itself is a potential means of grace, that it expresses a loving intention of which pregnancy and birth are the practical results.

In the language of the prologue to John's Gospel, the creative principle of the universe, the *logos*, was made flesh and dwells among us. Jesus Christ—who was from the beginning with God, by whom all things were made, and without whom "was not anything made that was made" (John 1:1-14)—is the crown and criterion of the mystery of God's creative love. Without presuming to know precisely *how* God creates, or for that matter *how* he is doing anything in the world, Christians nevertheless acknowledge and affirm *that* in God's action love accounts for creation and brings it into being. John 3:16, among other well-known passages, makes abundantly clear that it is out of God's love, and only because he loves, that he incarnates himself and thus establishes a certain loving relationship with the world. From this it follows that God creates nothing apart from his love and that incarnation is paradigmatic of authentic human relationships.

Christians have typically regarded the model of marriage and parenthood as that human relationship which most profoundly embraces and expresses this awareness; and this most succinctly explains why a Christian view of sex, marriage, and parenthood has never appropriately been preoccupied with ceremonies and conventions. What is important is whether a man and a woman pledge themselves to each other and consent to be responsible for each other; whether they consent together, witness the same, and pledge their fidelity to each other. When promise-making of this sort takes place between them, we rightly say that they love each other and imply that it is out of their love that they make these promises. If others, including clergymen, happen to be present when the couple articulates their marital intention in a public act, they only *witness* the marriage between these two. In the same way, law and custom may acknowledge marriage and exhibit it publicly. But a man and a woman marry each other.

Anyone who perceives and intends the world as a Christian will discover nothing new in this. Indeed, there are impressive sociological and psychological data, quite apart from any explicit Christian commitment, for the claim that love implies creation and vice-versa. Typically in our culture people fall in love and then have babies. We do not ordinarily have babies and then fall in love because, if in nothing more than inchoate awareness, we perceive a baby to be a special expression of an antecedent affection between those responsible for its being. But the obverse of this process is also at work: love wants to be particularized, concretized, incarnated; and people in love long for and self-consciously look for ways in which their love can be creative. Thus new beings like ourselves are procreated in the midst of our love for each other.

This dialectic is so fundamental to our *human* nature, as it were, that it seems inescapable: we procreate out of love because love requires it. To perceive and intend the world as Christians, that is, with reference to God's love incarnate as Jesus Christ, is to understand that love cannot escape responsibility for procreation and that procreation cannot authentically occur apart from love. Paul Ramsey has put the point plainly: "To put radically asunder what God joined together in parenthood when he made love procreative, to procreate from beyond the sphere of love . . . or to posit acts of sexual love beyond the sphere of responsible procreation (by definition, marriage), means a refusal of the image of God's creation in our own." [37] It is for this reason that the re-creational and procreative dimensions of human sexuality are finally inseparable. In certain intimate and intricate ways each depends upon the other for meaning, purpose, and value.

To speak this way about the inseparability of love-making and baby-making does not oblige us to insist that both must always be accomplished simultaneously. There are surely those times when couples appropriately and deliberately celebrate their love for each other sexually and without any *immediate* intention to procreate; just as, conversely, there are certainly those times (however rare!) when copulation is *immediately* decided by a temperature chart rather than a spontaneous and irrepressible erotic impulse. Still, human coition remains principally a single activity: its authenticity is more or less confirmed by (1) the *willingness* of both partners to incarnate their love in another human life, even when their intercourse is primarily unitive, and (2) their *intention* to surround new life, even when their intercourse is primarily procreative, with the love which unites them and longs for this embodiment. Every instance of coitus therefore need not intend procreation; on that point both Protestant and Catholic Christians agree.

There is, in this connection, a further question, and that is whether a couple might licitly adopt a lifelong policy of *un*parenthood in which the intention to procreate is not temporarily but permanently suspended. Again both Protestant and Catholic ethics allow for this exigency under certain circumstances—for example, reasonable fear of diseased children, economic disadvantage, and the like—but neither condones permanent unparenthood for mere expediency or convenience. Reasons for decisions of this sort finally reside deep in the hearts of those most immediately concerned, the couple themselves. They are free not to have children, although in doing so they must also forego a fulfillment that no other experience provides.

If we can begin to overcome the rooted cultural, religious, and philosophical traditions which locate *humanum* in one or another

---

[37] Paul Ramsey, "The Moral and Religious Implications of Genetic Control," in John Roslansky, ed., *Genetics and the Future of Man* (New York: Appleton-Century-Crofts, 1966), pp. 147-48.

kind of substance, we may begin to understand that we do not *have* sexuality in the sense that it is a possession to be kept or discarded. Whether to be a sexual creature is not an option. We *are* sexual creatures, and our sexuality is at least one of the ways in which we relate to each other at both superficial and profound levels of personal experience. To speak relationally about sexuality allows words like marriage, rape, adultery, and parenthood to take on distinctly *human* meaning; that is, what these and cognate words signify is a certain kind of relationship, or lack of it, between persons. What they mean is not adequate if limited to an objectification of behavior which limits and defines meaning with sole reference to overt action.

So we cannot any longer—if we ever could—speak of human sexuality as though it were merely a function of bodily metabolism. It is that, in part, but it is also a telos, an end in itself. Plants and animals exercise their sexuality, so far as we know, as merely natural phenomena; that is, they "throw off," as it were, objective evidence of themselves through sexual reproduction. But there may be at least this much difference between the sexual activity of persons and that of plants and animals: persons reproduce other unique, never-to-be-repeated persons. Persons incarnate their engendering love. Thus the sexual union of men and women is never a matter of simple reproduction or recreation; it is always an evidence, when it is authentic, of a loving relationship between them.

VI

The renowned American geneticist Hermann Joseph Muller once remarked that we are all fellow mutants together and that the only way to avoid ordinary, and thus more or less accidental, natural selection is by purposive control over human reproduction. If we translated Professor Muller's observation into theological language, we might say that we are all fellow creatures of this earth together, that we should responsibly control the human genetic pool, and that one of the marks of our moral maturity and responsibility is the manner in which we employ and limit, in intentional and purposive ways, the best methods available to us for establishing our proper dominion over the earth and advancing the quality of our common human life.

To put it this way is, of course, to reject the now discredited notion that nature's way is God's way and the similarly mistaken view that human mastery over human life processes verges on the demonic. Nothing in our experience is as readily apparent as change; and nothing in our religious awareness is as constant as the notion that change, inevitable as it seems to be, preferably takes place when directed by humane intelligence and moral sensitivity rather than when left to the caprice and whimsy of natural accident. The practical application of biomedical and bio-chemical investigations assumes that our species is not a com-pleted evolutionary product, either in the sense that it is without biological antecedents or that its present species characteristics are beyond improvement. It is arguable that the two-million-year evolution of our species as a humanly undirected process is near its end; at least we have at our disposal much of the technology, if not yet the wisdom, to direct evolution in ways that reflect our own intentions and purposes. No one yet claims to know what particular shape the future product ought to take, and it is that fact, together with our increasing capacity to control the process that produced us, that describes the moral dilemma of artificial insemination and genetic manipulation.

We will not get very far talking about the limits and obligations appropriate to the control of human life without some under-standing of words like *human, free, purposive,* and *responsible,* and the cultural and religious context out of which they come; but we presently appear to have achieved only vague consensus on these matters. A large part of our problem lies precisely in the fact that we have proceeded much faster and farther with scien-tific advance and technological sophistication than with meaning-ful networks of value within which our art and technics can re-sponsibly function. Fascination with experimentation, discovery, and innovation has outstripped our moral imagination, in conse-quence of which we find ourselves in the service of science and technology. It may be finally an article of faith, but I prefer to think that science and technology function best—that is, most appropriately and humanely—when they serve the needs and potentialities of human lives. Meantime, molecular biology and genetic engineering create new possibilities while we struggle to catch up with old accomplishments. Biomedical advance has usually proceeded with caution, and popular acceptance (as, for example, with blood transfusion) has come *ex post facto*. With the possibilities latent in manipulating genotypes we may very well have come to that point where we cannot wait upon the outcome before deciding whether the employment of this knowledge is good or bad. Some choices, however tentative and provisional, have to be made now. They carry with them, of course, an irreducible element of risk; but that seems to me morally preferable to abdication of deliberate choice to either natural determination or uncritical insistence on doing anything and everything which lies within our technical capability.

Approximately 500 defects are now suspected to be genetically controlled. We presently have only more or less effective tests, however, for fewer than 4 percent of these. Among the specific data now available, we know that 3 percent of the population carry the defective gene for cystic fibrosis, that 20 percent carry the defective gene for diabetes mellitus, that between 1 and 2 percent carry the defective gene for phenylketonuria (PKU). We know, moreover, that if a husband and wife have matching defective genes, the statistical chances are 1 in 4 that they will produce a defective child. Each of us, among our 10,000 to 100,000 genes, is likely to carry 5 to 10 defective genes; and that fact alone indicates how it is that 1 percent of live births are grossly defective, that another 1 percent are born with a defect serious enough to prevent marriage or holding a productive job, and that still another 4 to 6 percent of live births are abnormal in some way. Leroy Augenstein, a biophysicist who has given considerable attention to these matters, argues that things are getting worse, not better; and that because we are continuing to increase the pollution in our genetic pool, we can expect 10 percent of our children to be afflicted with a serious genetic defect within 75 to 150 years unless we begin now to cope with these problems.[38]

[38] Leroy Augenstein, *Come, Let Us Play God* (New York: Harper & Row, 1969), pp. 31-32.

According to Nobel Laureate Edward L. Tatum, three methods are currently proposed for modifying organisms and controlling our genetic future: eugenic engineering, genetic engineering, and euphenic engineering.[39] Eugenic engineering attempts a recombination of existing genes by directed control of conception through parental selection, artificial insemination, parthenogenesis, and the like. More specifically, this approach entails both negative eugenics (breeding *out* certain undesired genes as, for example, those responsible for retinoblastoma or diabetes mellitus) and positive eugenics (breeding *in* certain desired—but as yet unspecified—traits). Genetic engineering involves direct attack upon deleterious mutated genes by surgery or some anti-mutagent chemical which will cause genes to mutate back or be eliminated. Experiments utilizing this approach have thus far been almost entirely restricted to animals, micro-organisms, and viruses. Euphenic engineering undertakes to modify gene action in order to regulate certain deleterious effects of genetic disorder. Common examples of this method include insulin injections to compensate for inability to oxidize carbohydrate and gamma globulin injections to compensate for inability to synthesize this blood plasma protein. The relevant ethical questions directed to these methods have to do not only with means and ends, and the impressive social as well as private implications of such procedures, but also with those understandings of the nature and function of human sexuality which inform, and in some measure structure, human society.

I have argued that human procreation, Christianly understood, differs from animal or plant procreation precisely in the measure to which it functions within, and in order to incarnate, an antecedent loving relationship. I have argued, moreover, that on this understanding the two inseparable goods of human sexuality are disunited when procreation occurs from beyond the sphere of love or when acts of sexual love occur from beyond the sphere of willingness to be responsible for procreation.

In view of these arguments and the methods presently proposed

[39] Edward L. Tatum, "Perspectives From Physiological Genetics," in T. M. Sonneborn, ed., *The Control of Human Heredity and Evolution* (New York: The Macmillan Co., 1965), p. 22.

for control of our genetic future, direct attack upon dominant mutant genotypes—as, for example, the diseased hemoglobin which results in sicklecell anemia—though technically more difficult and less immediately feasible, is morally preferable to phenotypic breeding in or out of certain "desired" or "undesired" traits. Furthermore, it seems to me that negative (or preventive) eugenics can be recommended as a viable and licit undertaking, but that we should proceed cautiously—if at all!—with positive, or, as it is sometimes called, progressive, eugenics. In the long run—and given not only our technical capacity but also the moral sensibilities of our culture—I expect that euphenic biological engineering holds most promise and is most favorable to our direction of our evolution.

Glanville Williams' acerbic observation is worth quoting in this context. He says that "there is a striking contrast between human fecklessness in our own reproduction and the careful scientific improvement of other forms of life under man's control." [40] But this is a dare, for all the truth that's in it, that we cannot risk acting on; not least of all because human life, theologically perceived, is not properly subject to man in the same way as are other forms of life! Molecular biology, genetic manipulation, and other biomedical innovations *are* potential boons for the alleviation of some of our pains and fears; and they may help resolve some of our most vexing problems. But the opportunities they present are not unambiguously good; nor are all the implications yet known to us. What we urgently need is a sound philosophy of human life which will bring together the potential of molecular biology with other strands of human thought into a coherent and compassionate synthesis of human value. Meantime, it is appropriate for us to keep an eye on the distance between our technical sophistication and our moral sensibilities.

Because artificial insemination is already having broad effects in our social and political life, a judgment as to its morality deserves a reminder that words like adultery, parenthood, and legitimacy need not be the same in law as in theological ethics and morals. Neither Jesus' condemnation of divorce and remarriage

[40] *Sanctity of Life*, p. 82.

as adultery (Mark 10:11 and Luke 16:18), nor his reported saying that "whosoever looketh on a woman to lust after hath committed adultery with her already in his heart" (Matt. 5:28), is incorporated into the common law. The reasons for this are not our concern here; what is important is recognition that sin and crime are not synonymous categories and that a given action might appropriately be considered under one of these rubrics but not the other. This is, in fact, the case with AI: its legal status awaits determination with reference to the common good in a largely secular society. Meanwhile, Christians, Jews, and other religiously concerned citizens need to reflect on these issues from the perspective of particular theological and/or philosophical commitments; not because these reflections can or will be definitve in a pluralistic society, but because religious morality is one of the ingredients in the political and social mix.

The following observations are therefore formulated as provisional judgments about a modern human concern in the light of the church's teaching. This is not the last word, of course; but only the naïve and simple-minded will mistake an unwillingness to be definitive for an inability to be decisive. For the present, and in view of (1) the way Christians have understood sex and marriage, (2) what we now know about artificial insemination, and (3) other social and psychological factors which impinge upon this action, the most responsible (not to say the only) Christian response appears to be a qualified "yes" to AIH and a qualified "no" to AID.

In the case of AIH, there is no moral question of adultery inasmuch as the unitive and procreative dimensions of human sexuality are preserved. Moreover, a child thus conceived and born is in every sense truly the fruit of the union between *this* husband and wife who are parents both biologically and personally. As for the morality of the methods for securing the husband's semen, none is morally wrong *in principle*. Masturbation may be unpleasant or aesthetically objectionable, and if so there are several suitable (and, from a medical standpoint, perhaps even preferable) alternatives; but masturbation, in this context, may be licitly undertaken. In any case, it is a misnomer to label it "onanism."

Justification of AIH, however, cannot be unilaterally applied at every point to AID. AID separates procreation from love in the measure to which neither donor nor recipient posits his or her act within the sphere of a love which unites them. In AID each functions, as it were, from "outside" the other, thereby putting asunder "what God joined together" when he made love procreative.

To speak this way about AID is not to label it adultery. Indeed, AID is not adultery even in the conventional sense of being a deliberate and intentional carnal infidelity; the anonymity of the donor and the "impersonality" with which the operation is carried out sees to that. Neither is AID adultery in the sense of carnal lust (Matt. 5:28); what is sought in AID is not venereal pleasure, either actual or imagined, with another not one's spouse. Still, even with consent, AID signifies less than an unreserved commitment to share another's life "for better or worse, in sickness or in health."

It is the denial, however subtle, of this mutuality in marriage that shows how insidiously *hubris* can infect even our best intentions. So it is not lust in the conventional venereal sense, but lust in the sense of *envy* and *covetousness* that best characterizes the moral failure of AID. Why, it is argued, should a woman be deprived of the self-fulfillment of maternity just because she loves and is married to a man who happens to be sterile? I suggested earlier that the argument might just as compellingly be reversed: why should a man be deprived of the self-fulfillment of paternity just because he loves and is married to a woman who happens to be sterile? The answer lies, I think, in the ways that love and marriage qualify manhood and womanhood by husband-hood and wife-hood; which is only a shorthand way of saying that, by definition, personal fulfillment cannot be a private affair in the context of love and marriage, nor can it be achieved outside the sharing, involvement, and participation of the other.

In addition, we need to reexamine the popular assumption that parenthood is an inherent natural right. Obviously, in cases of natural sterility, it is not. But we are also learning from genetics, social psychology, and other relatively new disciplines that many factors impinge upon responsible parenthood. To cite only one example, I think it at least *arguable,* in view of the population explosion and a growing number of homeless and otherwise disadvantaged children, that AID is socially irresponsible and that adoption, which alleviates the needs of both childless couples and parentless children, offers a preferable alternative to involuntary childlessness.

No responsible person, to my knowledge, seriously argues that present population trends do not constitute a real and urgent problem. The annual net gain in United States population is now 2.6 million persons—an impressive figure in its own right, but one which achieves an almost incomprehensible magnitude when viewed in historical and archaeological perspective. It is estimated that between 800,000 and 1,000,000 years were required to bring the total number of human beings to 250 million by the beginning of the Christian era. Now *our* national net gain—to say nothing of the rest of the world—is annually at more than one tenth the total world population two thousand years ago!

For some time after the world's population reached 250 million, pestilence, disease, famine, and war kept the population increase down to only a fraction of 1 percent per year. In fact, sixteen centuries elapsed before the population doubled to 500 million. But 250 years later the world's population had reached 1 billion; less than a century later it was 2 billion; thirty years later it was 3 billion; by 1975, if net population increase continues at its present rate, it will be 4 billion; and in the next thirty years (i.e., by the year 2000) United Nations demographers estimate that the world's population will more than double, reaching approximately 6.9 billion persons. It is a sobering thought that *in about half a lifetime we will achieve a population increase that will exceed the total number of human beings produced in the one million years preceding the Christian era!*

It is this problem, some experts argue, and not the political embarrassments of Berlin or Vietnam that could trigger World War III—and particularly if the racial revolution focuses on the fact that it is the white man who has the food and the brown, black, and yellow men who have empty bellies.

The problem can be controlled in two ways: one way is by increasing the death rate, the other way is by decreasing the birthrate. It is not merely gratuitous to say that it is morally preferable to opt for decreasing the birthrate, even though nobody is seriously arguing for the other side (i.e., increasing the death rate). Given the value orientation of Western culture in general, and the Judeo-Christian tradition in particular, there are good and valid reasons for preferring lower birthrates to higher death rates. Among these is the claim that the entire family of man, as it is now constituted by the world's population, deserves to be respected and that no part of it can be treated callously or with personal disregard. Another principle, long honored and well known, perceives the difference between suicide and heroism and therefore encourages, as well as permits, acts of sacrificial service; so that childless couples might acknowledge and accept their inability to reproduce as a contribution to the common good. There are, of course, other social values which could be elicited; but the principal point need not be labored: given the demographic and ecologic facts of our time and place, adoption serves the common good better than AID.

Lastly, while courts and legislatures agonize about the legal responsibility of those who bring children into the world by AID, and the legitimacy of those thus born, there is no moral ambiguity as to the rights of AID babies. Of all parties, the child of AID is morally innocent of objections to this procedure because he has no responsible part in it; yet paradoxically, he is the only one who will bear in his person permanent existential reminder of the fact. There can be no reasonable doubt that however the legal questions are resolved, the AID child is morally entitled to every claim and benefit necessary and appropriate to his personal development and fulfillment.

One of the principal moral objections to AID would be overcome if the theoretical basis for progressive eugenics were perfected, but that is a dubious prospect because human genotypes are already so enormously varied. The magnitude of possible genotypes has been succinctly summarized by Bentley Glass:

The fertilized human egg contains 46 chromosomes, 23 of them inherited from the egg, 23 of them inherited from the sperm. The number of different genotypes that might be present in a single fertilized egg, if there were only 23 differences between the genes in the two sets of chromosomes in the father, and 23 other differences between the genes in the two sets of chromosomes in the mother, i.e., one difference per pair of chromosomes, would be $(2^{23})^2$. That is to say, the mother could potentially produce 2^{23}, or 8,388,608 genetically different sort of eggs, and the father an equal number of sperms with different genotypes. Hence there is a possibility through random fertilization of nearly 70 trillion genotypes of offspring. That would amount to about 2,300 generations of the entire present population of the entire world.[41]

The incredible mathematical possibility of gene combinations renders talk about "progressive eugenics" simplistic at the theoretical level. Beyond problems of this sort, however, we know very well that many other factors, in addition to genetic inheritance, play important roles in determining the shape and substance of human life. In terms of mere temporal expectation, it is not unlikely to suppose that we could improve human sociocultural conditions much more quickly than we can solve the theoretical and technical problems of eugenic engineering. Indeed, faced as we are with impressive social and cultural disadvantagement and accelerating crises from all sides, it is arguable that the highest priority belongs to these sociocultural matters.

Another lacuna might be bridged if the place of the family in Western civilization should give way to some other form of social organization. But still the onerous business, if genetic manipulation and AID are ever serious projects, of deciding what to breed for is inescapable: should it be for superior intellect, physical stamina and dexterity, moral goodness, or perhaps some combination of these and other ingredients? Even if these questions could be satisfactorily answered, someone would still need to show that all this would not sacrifice the person to the racial ambitions of a select few. What is ideal man? Who will decide? And how much experimental direct alteration of ecology, genotypes, and all the rest can we morally justify and humanly tolerate? Furthermore, should we not squarely face the question whether civilization as we know it could not be turned into madness; and the

[41] Bentley Glass, *Science and Ethical Values* (Chapel Hill: University of North Carolina Press, 1965), p. 40.

Christian faith as we know it replaced by an era which, through extreme depersonalization, would become genuinely *post mortem Dei?*

Especially since the time of the Enlightenment our (sometimes overwhelming) temptation has been to embrace every scientific and technological innovation because we suppose these things to be our salvation, to bring us closer to conquering the last remaining mystery of nature, and thus to assist us toward becoming entirely self-determining creatures. But discovery and mastery carry an increasing capacity for evil proportionate to the increasing capacity for good. Dean Inge once said that men who become wedded to the spirit of the times are likely to find themselves widowers in the next generation. The truth of that aphorism need not paralyze us, but it should appropriately give us pause.

III

Organ Transplantation and
Medical Experimentation

The end of life, like the beginning of it, occurs under a variety
of circumstances. Some persons die of generalized diseases, some
die violently, and some simply live so long that they just seem to
wear out. There are others who die because a particular part of
their body functions improperly or ceases to function at all. Until
recent years, recovery of persons in this latter category was predicated upon a fairly limited set of options: (1) the dysfunctional
or afunctional organ might spontaneously revive (sometimes assisted temporarily by supportive instrumentation);[1] (2) compen-
sation for dysfunction might be achieved with drugs (for example,
injection of insulin in cases of diabetes mellitus); or (3) a
mechanical appliance might be employed (for example, pace-

[1] Renal and peritoneal dialysis has sometimes functioned in this manner;
and it is interesting to note that one of the early experiences with kidney
transplantation ended with spontaneous recovery of the patient's own kidney
function. In 1949 Drs. Charles Hufnagel, Ernest Landsteiner, and David
Hume grafted a cadaveric kidney to the brachial artery and a large vein in
the antecubital fossa of a young woman suffering fron anuria. The cadaveric
kidney functioned for three days before it was removed (owing to decreasing
urine output and patient improvement). Dr. Hufnagel reported that "two or
three days after the removal of the kidney, the patient began to enter a
diuretic phase and her subsequent recovery was relatively uneventful." (Cited
in Francis D. Moore, *Give and Take—The Development of Tissue Transplantation* [Philadelphia: W. B. Saunders Co., 1964], pp. 14-15.)

makers in cases of cardiac arrhythmia). Now, however, increasing numbers of these patients have the remarkable additional possibility that tissue or whole organs may be transplanted into their bodies.

I

Historically, skin was the first tissue transplanted; and among the early experiments in this field were those carried out by Dr. Emile Holman in 1923-34. Holman's work suggested that recipients of skin grafts had the power to resist "foreign matter" in the form of grafts from donors and that an immune process of some sort was at work in graft rejection.[2] In the late 1920's, Dr. J. B. Brown of St. Louis and Dr. E. C. Padgett of Kansas[3] demonstrated that skin grafts between monozygotic twins could be successfully performed, thus suggesting that identical twins shared the same immune-response mechanism.

Neither of these discoveries, quite remarkable in retrospect, was generally appreciated, however, until two decades later when Professor Peter Medawar and his associates demonstrated that the destruction of foreign transplanted tissue is brought about by an active immunization mechanism in the recipient patient. More important, the Medawar group confirmed that the immunization mechanism "remembers" and "recognizes" alien tissues by describing and demonstrating the now well-known "second-set" rejection phenomenon; namely, that a second set of homografts (i.e., grafts from the same species, as opposed to heterografts, grafts from a different species) from the same donor to the same recipient will be rejected at an accelerated rate and thus more quickly than the first set.[4]

[2] Emile Holman, "Protein sensitization in isoskingrafting. Is the latter of practical value?" *Surgery, Gynecology, and Obstetrics* (1924), 38:100. This process, incidentally, is still being investigated by immunologists because it is now, more than ever before, thought to be the key to transplantation compatibility.

[3] J. B. Brown, "Homografting of skin: with report of success in identical twins," *Surgery* (1937), 1:558; E. C. Padgett, "Is iso-skin grafting practicable?" *Southern Medical Journal* (1932), 25:895.

[4] P. B. Medawar, "The behavior and fate of skin autografts and skin

Almost ten years later Medawar and his colleagues published the results of their work toward overcoming immune reactions and inducing an "actively acquired tolerance" in recipients for homografts. The procedure was to inject foreign cells into very young animals whose response to them was inverted; instead of acquiring an immune reaction, these animals acquired a tolerance for these cells, and foreign tissue of that same type could then be grafted to them without rejection.[5] Despite the inapplicability of this procedure to human beings,[6] it had now been demonstrated that the barrier to tissue transplantation was not insurmountable.

Meanwhile, experiments with renal, or kidney, homografts and heterografts in animals were perfecting the technical surgical aspects of this operation. In this context, the work of Drs. Alexis Carrel and Carl F. Williamson in the United States, Dr. Morton Simonsen in Copenhagen, and Dr. William Dempster in London deserves special mention. At about the same time, Dr. Willem Kolff was developing the first successful artificial kidney. Working secretly under the handicap of Nazi occupation of Holland, Kolff fabricated a machine which could dialyze the blood of a patient afflicted with chronic kidney disease and wash away the accumulated urea.[7]

homografts in rabbits" (a report to the War Wounds Committee of the Medical Research Council), *Journal of Anatomy* (1944), 78:176. See also P. B. Medawar, "A second study of the behavior and fate of skin homografts in rabbits" (a report to the War Wounds Committee of the Medical Research Council), *Journal of Anatomy* (1945), 79:157.

[5] R. E. Billingham, L. Brent, and P. B. Medawar, " 'Actively acquired tolerance' of foreign cells," *Nature* (1953), 172:603.

[6] Professor Michael Woodruff and his colleagues demonstrated the technical feasibility of the procedure in humans, but abandoned further research because of potential dangers to subjects. M. F. A. Woodruff and L. O. Simpson, "Induction of tolerance to skin homografts in rats by injection of cells from the prospective donor soon after birth," *British Journal of Experimental Pathology* (1955), 36:494; and M. F. A. Woodruff, "Can tolerance to homologous skin be induced in the human infant at birth?" *Transplantation Bulletin* (1957), 4:26. As recently as March, 1969, at a conference on biology and transplantation in Glasgow, Scotland, the suggestion was put forward that intraplacental injection may be the solution to immunological problems!

[7] W. J. Kolff and H. Th. J. Berk, "The artificial kidney: a dialyser with a great area," *Acta Medica Scandinavica* (1944), 117:121; and W. J. Kolff,

These events, together with others too numerous to cite here, laid the foundations for the first experiments with homografts in human beings. Following a series of unsuccessful kidney transplantations between unrelated donors and recipients and without immuno-suppression, the first successful human renal homograft was carried out between adult identical twins in 1954 by Dr. Joseph E. Murray and his associates at Boston's Peter Bent Brigham Hospital. By 1958 the Brigham team had done seven kidney isotransplants, i.e., using identical twins, of which three failed;[8] and in 1959 Murray's group performed the first successful human homograft between other than monozygotic twins, using dizygotic or fraternal twins and total body irradiation to surmount the moderate immunological barrier.[9] Two years yater Murray and his colleagues successfully employed azathioprine, an immuno-suppressive drug, to combat rejection for thirty-six days; and in important ways this feat marks the present state of organ (and especially kidney) transplantation with its widespread use of a variety of drugs which enable the homograft to survive without destroying or seriously jeopardizing the recipient's immunological mechanism.[10]

The recipient of the 1954 transplant died eight years later of coronary artery disease and glomerulonephritis in the transplanted

---

New Ways of Treating Uraemia; The Artificial Kidney, Peritoneal Lavage, Intestinal Lavage (London: W. & M. Churchill, 1947).

[8] J. E. Murray, J. P. Merrill, and J. H. Harrison, "Kidney transplantation between seven pairs of identical twins," *Annals of Surgery* (1958), 148:343.

[9] J. E. Murray, J. P. Merrill, G. J. Dammin, J. B. Dealy, C. W. Walter, M. S. Brooke, and R. E. Wilson, "Study of transplantation immunity after total body irradiation: clinical and experimental investigation," *Surgery* (1960), 48:272.

[10] The four drugs most commonly used for immuno-suppression in homo-transplants are actinomycin, azaserine, cortisone, and 6-mercaptopurine (to which azathioprine is closely related). While different, they appear to achieve largely the same result. The patient who survived for thirty-six days with azathioprine died, ironically, of toxicity induced by the administration of that same drug. Clinicians now employ fairly precise parameters for determining the optimum use of these drugs. See J. E. Murray, J. P. Merrill, J. H. Harrison, R. E. Wilson, and G. J. Dammin, "Prolonged survival of human kidney homografts by immunosuppressive drug therapy," *New England Journal of Medicine* (1963), 268:1315.

kidney. That first case in the series is important not only because it was a breakthrough in medical technology and surgical technique, but also because it propounded a moral dilemma which is still only cautiously resolved in cases which involve transplanting a paired organ from a living donor: Is it ever right or proper to take a normal organ from a healthy person in order to replace a diseased organ in a sick person? That question was largely avoided in early clinical experience because human renal homotransplants had been performed with kidneys from cadaveric donors or those necessarily removed during therapeutic surgery (the so-called "free organs" secured, for example, from operations for ureteral cancer, or the creation of a subarachnoid-ureteral shunt). Now, however, with some knowledge of the immune-response mechanism and the technical sophistication needed to do human homografts, the morality of one person suffering bodily mutilation for the benefit of another became an explicit issue.

We have so far focused attention on kidney transplantation because of its role in the genesis of human homotransplantation. Not only were renal homografts the first successfully performed human transplants; they have also been the subject of most of the specifically forensic opinions that are presently available. Skin, artery, bone, and cornea were transplanted prior to kidneys; but these, with the exception of skin grafts, are more on the order of *homostructural grafts* than homotransplants, and, moreover, they do not excite a destructive immune response. It is arguable, of course, that some of the basic issues posed by organ transplantation were implied, if not seriously recognized or acknowledged, in the initial employment of prostheses for human beings; and that extracting or repairing teeth, or fitting a person with dentures or inlays, already raised questions about bodily integrity, mutilation, and totality. The fact is, however, that these questions lay largely dormant for many centuries and became active issues only with the advent of human renal homografts. Still, concern about these things, even at this stage, was relegated to a relative few among both the medical profession and the lay public until December 3, 1967, when, for the first time, a human heart was transplanted into a human body.

II

Prior to the first human heart homograft, to be sure, a great deal of research and operating technique had been developed in cardiac surgery. In fact, almost four years earlier, in January, 1964, Dr. James D. Hardy and his associates in Mississippi had made an unsuccessful attempt at heart heterotransplantation. The donor in this case was a chimpanzee and the recipient a sixty-eight-year-old man suffering from hypertensive cardiovascular disease. Hardy acknowledged that there were problems associated with a procedure of this sort: "The clinical transplantation of a human heart might prompt controversy, and the clinical transplantation of the primate heart was even more likely to arouse controversy. Even so, it was felt that to perform this transplant, under the specific set of circumstances which existed at that instant, was well within ethical and moral boundaries." [11] Just where those boundaries are, or were, was not described by Hardy; and one can only speculate about what he had in mind, or whether his statement was merely polite acknowledgment that this was at best a borderline case.

Toward the end of Hardy's published report there are three paragraphs under the heading "Moral Issue of Clinical Heart Transplantation" which defend this action as the patient's only chance for survival. Overall, it was a very poor chance indeed. According to the same report, the patient was admitted to the surgical service with gangrene of the lower left leg and a long history of hypertensive cardiovascular disease; he was in a stuporous or semicomatose condition, suffering from atrial fibrillation, and registering a fluctuating blood pressure at a systolic level of between 90 and 110 mm Hg.; his respiratory effort was so inadequate that a tracheostomy and mechanical ventilatory assistance were required; both lower extremeties were edematous and the lower left leg was amputated; the cardiologist's conclusion was that the patient was unequivocally critical due to myocardial failure and

[11] James D. Hardy, Carlos M. Chavez, Fred D. Kurrus, William A. Neely, Sadan Eraslan, M. Don Turner, Leonard W. Fabian, and Thaddeus D. Labecki, "Heart Transplantation in Man: Developmental Studies and Report of a Case, *Journal of the American Medical Association* (1964), 188:1132-40. It is of incidental interest in this context to note that a sheep's heart was used in a heterotransplant in 1968; it also failed. (*Time*, December 6, 1968.)

multiple emboli; he was sixty-eight years old. It is hardly surprising in view of these factors, together with the uncertainties of a heterotransplant, that the patient died shortly over an hour after mechanical support was withdrawn.

There is no mention in the report that adequate consent had been obtained. And there is evidence that news releases were ineptly managed; in fact, the hospital authorities appear to have suppressed information about the operation until staff leakages made this no longer possible. It is doubtless arguable that these latter considerations are collateral issues; still, they confirm and give additional weight to the judgment that *in this case* the limits of human experimental protocols were exceeded. In the end, the expectation that transplantation of a primate heart would arouse more controversy than transplantation of a human heart was not fulfilled; there was no public outcry and only modest professional notice, and almost four years passed before the Washkansky case catapulted heart transplantation into international prominence.

Enough experimentation had taken place by 1967 to demonstrate that transplantation of the heart is a relatively simple operation *mechanically*. The preferred surgical techniques for the four major anastamoses were developed by 1959, and successful homotransplantation of the heart in dogs was reported as early as 1962.[12] In 1966 Dr. Joseph Murray, whose group had performed the first successful human renal homotransplant, suggested that "the heart is a feasible organ to transplant because its function is really less complex than that of other tissues, as it is principally a pump and consists of tissues from one germinal source." Moreover, he added that "heart tissue is probably less antigenic than epithelial tissue." [13] The immune-response mechanism, however, continues to plague transplantation and make it significantly more than a mere mechanical procedure.

[12] R. R. Lower, R. C. Stofer, E. J. Hurley, E. Dong, Jr., R. B. Cohn, and N. E. Shumway, "Successful Homotransplantation of the Canine Heart After Anoxic Preservation for Seven Hours," *American Journal of Surgery* (1962), 104:302.

[13] Joseph E. Murray, "Organ Transplantation: The Practical Possibilities," in *Ethics in Medical Progress*, ed. G. E. W. Wolstenholme and Maeve O'Connor (Boston: Little, Brown, 1966), p. 64.

On December 3, 1967, Dr. Christiaan Barnard and his team at the Groote Schuur Hospital in Cape Town, South Africa, performed the first human heart transplant. The donor was twenty-five-year-old Denise Darvall, who had been admitted to the hospital on December 2 with what was described as irreversibly fatal brain damage resulting from an automobile accident. The recipient was Louis Washkansky, a fifty-five-year-old diabetic with a history of coronary artery disease and two heart attacks within seven years. News of Barnard's feat immediately captured worldwide attention: newspapers carried banner headlines reading "Heart Transplant Success," magazines described it as "the ultimate operation," [14] and at least one doctor ventured the opinion that Washkansky stood "quite a definite chance" of surviving the transplant "at least two years or more." [15] Other physicians were somewhat more cautious. Dr. Michael DeBakey, himself a distinguished cardiovascular surgeon, was quoted as saying that the transplant "certainly would be a great achievement if they'll be able to overcome the rejection." [16] For almost three weeks an anxious and curious world received regular hospital bulletins. Eighteen days after the operation Washkansky died. While the possibility of rejection was not excluded, the autopsy report released by Barnard attributed death to "respiratory failure due to bilateral pneumonia."

In retrospect, and apart from the purely surgical aspects of the case, at least two factors in the Washkansky case merit more serious consideration than they received in December, 1967: the operation was undertaken without white blood cell matching and on a patient known to be already afflicted with diabetes.[17] The time element was undoubtedly a critical factor in this operation. White cell matching can be a long and complicated process with cells from the same person alternating among the known twenty-three types within only a few hours. Despite the fact that Miss

[14] *Time*, December 15, 1967.
[15] Dr. Kenneth Sell, quoted in an Associated Press dispatch by science writer Frank Carey, December 4, 1967.
[16] Quoted by Alton Blakeslee and John Barbour in an Associated Press Dispatch, December 4, 1967.
[17] See *Time*, December 15, 1967. In addition, Washkansky's liver was enlarged and he was edematous.

Darval's heart was being perfused with oxygenated blood in anticipation of the transplant, white cell matching may have been infeasible; but none of the reports of the operation suggest *why* there was no time to assess tissue compatibility. In view of what was then known about immune-response mechanisms, blood cell and tissue typing, the observation of a Soviet doctor stated the crux of the matter: "Even if such an operation is successful, the success would be accidental." [18]

The second factor relates to the first in that there is an established deleterious relationship between diabetes and steroids such as those employed in immuno-suppressive drugs. Since the recipient would be subjected to massive dosages of radiation and immuno-suppressive therapy (in Washkansky's case, azathioprine [imuran] and cortisone) in an effort to combat the rejection mechanism, it is reasonable to suppose that the chances of viral infection were increased and the prospect for survival correspondingly diminished. Beyond this, Washkansky was not restricted to an aseptic environment. Moreover, there is some evidence for suspecting that long-term recipients of immuno-suppressive drugs are liable to a higher than usual incidence of malignancy.

In defense of the operation, and like the earlier Hardy case, Barnard stated in an article "especially written" for the Associated Press that Washkansky's disease was "incurable by any known treatment other than cardiac transplantation." [19] Without quibbling over semantics and whether heart transplantation could be accurately described as a "known treatment" before it was attempted, a comment from John Lear's perceptive critique pinpoints a further problematic factor in the decision to remove the heart of a coronary artery disease victim:

[18] Associated Press, December 22, 1967.
[19] Associated Press, December 11, 1967. A few weeks later one of my students reported that he had had opportunity to talk briefly with Barnard in Houston, Texas, and that he had asked the surgeon whether he (Barnard) attached any theological significance to heart transplantation. According to the student, Barnard's response was a spontaneous recitation of Ezekiel 11:19 ("And I will give them one heart, and I will put a new spirit within you; and I will take the stony heart out of their flesh, and will give them an heart of flesh.")! This is not the place to assess Barnard's exegesis of Ezekiel; on the other hand, it might not be inappropriate to wish that more theologians were similarly well versed in the literature of medicine.

97

Thousands of people are walking around, some of them working strenuously, with hearts that have been on the verge of collapse for years. To remove one of those apparently faltering pumps amounts to substitution of a statistical certainty for a statistical uncertainty. The statistical certainty is that a transplant recipient, in the present state of knowledge about the body's immunological system, will lose to infection or rejection within a year and a half at most, probably much sooner.[20]

Neither Lear's point nor the earlier observations on this case are intended to question the motives or technical skill of the team that operated on Washkansky, and that should be clearly understood. What is at issue is whether *in this case* and others like it the odds were too heavily against success in a decision to transplant. The greater weight of the evidence suggests that they were. Indeed, the predictable chances for survival have been poor in virtually all the heart transplantations undertaken thus far; and some of them (for example, the case of Michael Kasperak) have been attended by such heroic and extraordinary measures as to evoke public criticisms from doctors themselves.[21]

Well over a hundred human heart transplants had been performed by the spring of 1969, when worldwide press notices gave frontpage coverage to the case of Haskell Karp in Houston, Texas. On April 4, Good Friday in the Christian liturgical year, Karp was the recipient of what was termed the "first total replacement of a human heart by a mechanical device." [22] The surgery was performed by Dr. Denton Cooley, who has done more of these operations than any other surgeon, and its purpose was admittedly a temporary expedient until a donor could be found for a homograft. After an emotion-packed nationwide appeal by Karp's wife —carried also by overseas television networks—a donor was secured and the transplant immediately performed on April 7. Karp died the following day. The announcement from St. Luke's Hospital stated that "it is suspected that the patient suffered acute rejection complicated by pneumonia and kidney failure." [23] Again it is

[20] Lear, "Transplanting the Heart," *Saturday Review*, January 6, 1968.
[21] Associated Press dispatch, January 23, 1968.
[22] Reuter news dispatch, April 5, 1969.
[23] Reuter news dispatch, April 9, 1969.

difficult not to think, in view of what is now known about immune-response mechanisms and the long and complicated processes necessary for cell matching and tissue typing, that the speed with which this particular transplant proceeded from donor to recipient foreclosed serious promise of long-term success. And the question once more is simply whether, in this and similar cases, there can be *reasonable* expectation that the operation will provide real therapeutic benefit to the patient.[24]

III

Immunological incompatibilities between donor and recipient are generally regarded as the most important single factor in accounting for transplant failure, and the selection of a compatible donor would therefore seem to be the most basic step toward preventing rejection.[25] Odds are presently about 100 to 1 that a recipient will get a tissue type that exactly matches his own. In view of this fact, it would further appear that exclusive preoccupa-

[24] Dr. Eugene D. Robin headed a list of seven considerations that should apply in human homotransplantation with the proposition that the transplant should have some reasonable possibility of clinical success and only be undertaken with an acceptable therapeutic goal as its purpose. Eugene D. Robin, "Rapid Scientific Advances Bring New Ethical Questions," *Journal of the American Medical Association* (1964), 189:112-3.

[25] Delford L. Stickel, *Ethical and Moral Aspects of Transplantation* (Monographs in the Surgical Sciences," Vol. III, No. 4; Baltimore: The Williams & Wilkins Co., 1966), p. 270. See also J. E. Murray, R. Gleason, and A. Bartholomay, "Fourth Report of the Human Kidney Transplant Registry: 16 Sept. 1964 to 15 March 1965," *Transplantation* (1965), 3:684; and P. S. Russell and A. P. Monaco, "The Biology of Tissue Transplantation," *New England Journal of Medicine* (1964), 271:502. Experience with kidney transplantation indicates that the one-year survival rate for recipients of renal homografts is about 80 percent with close relative donors, about 60 percent with cadaveric donors, and less than 30 percent with living unrelated donors. In this context, it is further instructive to note that the increased mortality risk to living donors (i.e., in having one normal kidney instead of two) for the five years following nephrectomy is anticipated at 99.1 percent as compared with a normal expectation of 99.3 percent (a risk comparable to that of a commuter who travels 16 miles per working day or less than 8,000 miles per year.) Cf. J. P. Merrill, "Clinical Experience Is Tempered by Genuine Human Concern," *Journal of the American Medical Association* (1964), 189:114.

tion with recipients is not calculated to achieve the best surgical results. It is entirely understandable that confrontation with a patient's urgent need for organ replacement evokes the doctor's deep and irrepressible human concern to do all within his power immediately to meet that need. On the other hand, there is a moral as well as scientific obligation to employ those limited organs that are available for transplantation to the best possible advantage.

Given the dearth of viable organs for transplantation and the difficulty with which they are usually secured, it would constitute better stewardship of the organs and better faith with their donors if the priorities were slightly altered, as they have been by some transplant teams; that is, instead of making the decision chiefly with reference to a patient's need for *a transplant,* the choice of recipient should be made on the basis of immunologic compatibility with *the available organ.* Because the demand for organs far exceeds their supply, to proceed this way would require only that adequate time be secured for typing and matching. Prototype "organ preservation chambers" have already been developed and used experimentally, and there is every reason to expect that such instrumentation may become functional in the near future. Meantime, what is already common practice in heart and other unpaired organ transplantation—namely, perfusing a corpse with oxygenated blood between pronouncement of death and transplantation—can be extended, at least for a while, in order to establish better immunologic compatibility with the prospective recipient(s).[26]

This may appear to be a harsh and insensitive approach, but it is in fact no different from those other hard choices which are forced upon us by as yet limited resource and inadequate information. One of the dramatic, but by no means unique, instances of this sort occurs with the comparatively small number of dialysis units available for the thousands of patients who suffer from

[26] Apart from logistical questions regarding the adequacy of apparatus, space, personnel, and the like, there are other problems (which we will discuss in the next chapter) which have to do with the criteria and definition of death in view of the technical capacity to extend certain vital life processes, particularly respiration and circulation, almost indefinitely.

chronic kidney failure. When it became generally known in 1962 that Seattle's Artificial Kidney Center at Swedish Hospital was selecting candidates for renal dialysis on a broader basis than immediate and urgent need, both professional and public response ranged from outrage to admiration. Some said that the committee, appointed by the county Medical Society, was making decisions of life and death that they had no moral and humane right to make; others maintained, in view of many claims upon few machines, that the committee was performing a responsible and unavoidable (however onerous) duty both to the individual candidates and the larger society. The committee itself recognized the moral ambiguity of decisions and that a number of serious risks were involved in their choices. Still, they elected to exercise their limited freedom in the light of their best understanding. Nobody can be asked to do more than that; and that their choices did not always result in unambiguously good results may be credited more to creatureliness than a bad will or defective conscience. Now, under somewhat similar circumstances, increasing numbers of surgeons are refusing to perform renal transplants—even when this decision virtually assures the death of a patient—when an immunologically compatible donor organ is not available. Again, a cluster of values occurring in a particular mix shapes decisions of this sort: concern for patient well-being, use of the donor organ, conservation of resources, deployment of personnel, utilization of hospital facilities, cost, and many others. The point, withal, is that the well-being of a particular transplant candidate, when understood as something more than mere life-prolongation, may sometimes constrain a surgeon to decide *not to transplant* an available organ which is immunologically incompatible with that patient.[27]

[27] In February, 1964, Dr. J. R. Elkington wrote an editorial in the *Annals of Internal Medicine* (60:309-13) entitled, "Moral Problems in the Use of Borrowed Organs, Artificial and Transplanted." An enormous correspondence was evoked by this piece and in the August, 1964, issue of the journal, Elkington undertook to summarize the areas of agreement and disagreement reflected in communications. The first two of five summary statements, interestingly, include the following: "Compassionate concern for the patient as a total person is the primary goal of the physician and the investigator—*on this point all agree*. . . . Violation of the personality and iden-

During the 12 months which followed the epoch-making Washkansky operation, 95 human hearts were transplanted into 93 patients (two patients received two hearts each) at 36 medical centers in 16 countries. In December, 1968, less than half those patients were living (some had only recently been transplanted) and another death among their number was being regularly reported. By August, 1969, the statistics disclosed that of at least 142 cardiac homografts performed in the 20 months following the initial transplant, 37 patients were still alive. And by June, 1970, only 10 survivors remained of more than 160 heart transplantations.[28]

If one grants, as I think we must, that doctors, like the rest of us, are not wholly immune to certain pressures that ordinarily have little to do with the exercise of purely professional roles, the part that mass media has played in this brief history of organ transplantation (and particularly heart transplantation) surely cannot be ignored. It is difficult, perhaps even impossible, to document the precise ways in which news reporting has contributed to the public clamor for more, and more daring, feats of surgical experimentation and innovation; nevertheless, some things are fairly clear. Dr. Barnard and his team, to their credit, were apparently quite open with reporters and withheld little if any information of consequence in the Washkansky case. Still, news stories at that time did not tell the full story; even worse, their sometimes melodramatic and overly optimistic reports gave false hopes to thousands of heart disease patients. That unrestrained

---

tity of the recipient would occur only with transplantation of the brain; this is not a hazard in the foreseeable future. *But it is the ultimate moral danger of the artificial reconstruction of living human bodies by other human beings.*" See *Annals of Internal Medicine* (1964), 61:363.

[28] The most conspicuous success to date has been Louis B. Russell, Jr., a 45-year-old schoolteacher from Indianapolis, who received his transplant on August 24, 1968, in Richmond's Medical College of Virginia. As of mid-summer, 1970, Russell was reported to be robust and healthy. The previous record for heart transplant survival was set by Philip Blaiberg, who died 594 days post-transplant. In January, 1969, Dr. Barnard told a world conference on death and reanimation that present techniques have achieved good results and that "the possibility of success, in fact, has risen to about 35 percent." (*The Scotsman*, Edinburgh, January 14, 1969.) There remains, however, a question about the meaning of "success," and to the present time, at least, a statistical gap between this possibility and the realities of heart transplantation.

enthusiasm bordering on irresponsibility created something like a carnival atmosphere at the Groote Schuur Hospital is attested in part by the fact that at least one camera crew surreptitiously gained access to Barnard's operating theater.

Beyond violations of this sort, one might point to the contradiction of giving front-page coverage, sometimes with pictures, of dramatic surgical exploits and then ignoring or burying unobtrusively news of failure and death; or to the uncritical use of extravagant words like "breakthrough" and "treatment" to describe procedures that are frankly experimental;[29] or to the plight of surgeons involved in such notoriety who are subsequently inundated by requests from patients for the same operation. It was generally known that twenty or more surgical teams throughout the world were poised ready to perform the first human heart transplant when the right conditions occurred; and it is more than an idle question whether—and if so, to what extent—journalistic sensationalism contributed to the uncommonly large number (some quite untimely) of heart transplantations which immediately followed Barnard's initial operation.

Doctors themselves, together with laboratory investigators, are not altogether blameless in this. They must bear final responsibility for their professional decisions despite the coercive power of news media; indeed, they are the first to insist upon having it no other way. Nevertheless, awareness of some of the kinds of pressure to which they are subjected, among them public opinion and the ways in which it is molded, makes some of their actions more understandable, if not more justifiable. The decisional apparatus of doctors (no less than the rest of us) is, after all, not entirely described by an insular professionalism; and the role of the press and other instruments of modern mass communications therefore requires a heightened sense of responsibility and discretion. Perhaps the crux of the matter, as it bears upon news coverage, was suitably summed up in a one-liner from a member of the British Parliament who rebutted a colleague's speech by saying, "Sir, we are entitled to the correct version of the truth."

[29] Cf. Irvine H. Page, editorial, "Unwise Publicity," *Modern Medicine*, January 20, 1964, pp. 81 ff.

IV

Legal reflections upon organ transplantation have focused, perhaps understandably, more extensively upon the donor than upon the recipient, and more directly upon renal than other types of homografting. There tends to be a presumption among lawyers and jurists that the recipient's rights are *de facto* protected by the curative or therapeutic character of the procedure itself. And although informed and voluntary consent from the patient is commonly indispensable for every type of surgical procedure, it is argued by some that a transplant recipient's formal consent may not be required under certain extenuating circumstances. For example, Professor David Daube has maintained that "an unconscious adult should be given a transplantation he needs unless we know that he does not want it: there is no difference here from an ordinary operation. Again, a minor should be given a transplantation if the doctors deem it necessary, even against the will of the parents." [30] The late Professor Alexander Kidd was more cautious:

In general, a medical man may not treat or operate on a human being without his consent. It makes no difference that the person needs treatment or will die if he does not get it. If the consent has not been obtained, it is no defense that the operation was skillfully performed and saved the patient's life. Where the patient is unconscious and needs immediate treatment, it can be done; but even there, if the husband or wife is present, his or her consent may be necessary. [31]

If the principle of the "greater weight of evidence" applies to this argument, it is probably fair to conclude that the legal problems most generally pertinent to transplantation are those having to do with consent by the donor or those authorized by law to speak in his behalf.

In the Ciba Foundation symposium, *Ethics in Medical Progress*, Professor David Louisell discussed the legal aspects of con-

---

[30] David Daube, "Transplantation: Acceptability of Procedures and the Required Legal Sanctions," in *Ethics in Medical Progress*, pp, 196-97.

[31] Alexander M. Kidd, "Limits of the Right of a Person to Consent to Experimentation on Himself," *Science* (1953), 117:211-12.

sent and transplantation in terms of living persons, cadavers, and what he aptly called the "twilight zone." [32] According to Louisell, there is no serious legal problem where both the donor and recipient are competent adults who give informed and voluntary consent.[33] But responsibility for obtaining that consent is vested in the physician, and failure to secure it may make him "liable for battery, assault if the patient is conscious, or for negligence for failure to communicate with his patient with reasonable care." [34]

Under common law all minors are held to be incapable of giving valid consent, and therefore the explicit consent of parents or guardians is usually required. In the case of operations which are clearly for the child's benefit, there is no commonsense reason to repudiate the adequacy of parental consent under common law. But where the procedure poses only risk to the child and benefit to another, the situation is significantly altered, and serious questions arise with respect to whether anybody, adult or child, can legitimately give consent for a minor to become an organ donor. The most significant opinions thus far are contained in three declaratory judgments of the Supreme Judicial Court of Massachusets,[35] which were given at the initiative of the surgical staff and trustees of Peter Bent Brigham Hospital. Following its successful experience with the 1954 kidney transplantation between adult identical twins, the hospital had received a number of requests for the same operation on identical twins who were minors.

In 1956 three cases—two involving fourteen-year-old twins and the other nineteen-year-old twins—were presented as potential candidates for renal homotransplantation. Each case was heard before a different justice of the court and each justice wrote an individual opinion. The three opinions were almost identical, and in each instance the operation was allowed. In sum, four ingredi-

[32] David W. Louisell, "Transplantation: Existing Legal Constraints," in *Ethics in Medical Progress*, pp. 80-94.

[33] Cf. I. Packel, "Spare Parts for the Human Engine," *Pennsylvania Bar Association Quarterly* (1965), 37:71 ff.

[34] Louisell, in *Ethics in Medical Progress*, p. 83. Cf. W. L. Prosser, *Torts*, (3rd ed.; St. Paul: West Publishing Co., 1964), pp. 104-6.

[35] Masden v. Harrison, No. 68651 Eq., Mass. Sup. Jud. Ct., June 12, 1957; Huskey v. Harrison, No. 68666 Eq., Mass. Sup. Jud. Ct., Aug. 30, 1957; Foster v. Harrison, No. 68674 Eq., Mass. Sup. Jud. Ct., Nov. 20, 1957.

ents were prominent in the three judgments: (1) consent of the parents; (2) necessity of the operation to save the sick twin; (3) understanding of the operation and voluntary consent by the healthy twin; and (4) psychiatric testimony that the operation was necessary for the continued good health and future well-being of the *donor*.

More recently, in a case involving adult siblings in Kentucky, the same reasoning, with the conspicuous exception of the third ingredient, was employed to authorize a renal transplant.[36] Jerry Strunk was judged by doctors to be the best kidney donor for his brother, Tommy. Jerry was confined to a state mental hospital and mentally incompetent to give valid consent. The mother of the boys favored the operation and asked a court to authorize it. Jerry's state-appointed guardian, however, objected. The Kentucky Court of Appeals nevertheless upheld the decision of a lower court to approve the transplant on the ground that Jerry's well-being "would be jeopardized more severely by the loss of his brother than the removal of a kidney." Unique to this case is the mental incompetence of the donor; in the Massachusetts cases it was argued that minors had understood and given voluntary consent to being donors. There is not, however, that much to commend the Kentucky decisions; and otherwise generally unsubstantiated fears of recapitulating the Nazi atrocities in modern experimental procedures are given support by such shallow reasoning and overt circumvention of both the spirit and letter of the law.

Commenting upon the Massachusetts cases, William J. Curran has raised several provocative questions; among them whether the psychiatric opinion that the healthy twin would suffer a "grave emotional impact on the death of his twin brother" deserves to be treated as more than common sense; why, in view of the common law, the court should require not only parental consent but also consent of each of the twins as well; and why the justices did not squarely face the issues posed by lack of direct therapeutic benefit to the healthy twin? [37]

These queries are to the point and warrant sober reflection.

[36] "A Brother's Sacrifice," *Time*, November 7, 1969.

[37] William J. Curran, "A Problem of Consent: Kidney Transplantation in Minors, *New York University Law Review* (1959), 34:891-98.

That the two fourteen-year-olds who received their twins' kidneys died within some months of the operations does nothing to diminish or detract from the seriousness of Curran's implied criticisms. It makes sense that the psychiatric testimony was merely common sense in technical jargon and that judgments which fail to face squarely the fundamental issues hold little promise of becoming precedents. In the present situation, Daube's proposal is perhaps the most prudent: he advocates extending the age of consent downward "to roughly the age of conscription," but not compromising it in any case. Thus, the alleged likelihood of psychological trauma in situations like those described above "will be greatly lessened if the law leaves not the shadow of a doubt that a transplantation is here out of the question: the case will then be no different from where a twin dies from pneumonia —bad enough, but with no scope for offer of a sacrifice, disappointment, self-torture." [38]

Cadaveric organs, like those of living donors, are legally available for transplantation if requirements for proper authorization and consent are fulfilled. Half a century ago Justice Cardozo enunciated the principle that "every human being of adult years and sound mind has a right to determine what shall be done with his own body," [39] and present common law, except as modified by statute, continues to affirm that right. In the event that a decedent has not made specific and valid provision for disposition of his body, the right of possession typically belongs (respectively) to the surviving spouse, children, or next of kin. [40] Louisell points out that where the decedent has made no provision for disposal of his body, including the donation of organs, physicians may avoid criminal or civil liability for mutilating a corpse by obtaining the consent of those legally entitled to the body before removing organs. [41]

[38] Daube, in *Ethics in Medical Progress*, p. 198.

[39] *Schloendorff* v. *New York Hospital*, 211 N. Y. 125, 105 N. E. 92 (1914).

[40] Cf. A. D. Vestal, R. E. Taber, and W. J. Shoemaker, "Medical-Legal Aspects of Tissue Homotransplantation," *University of Detroit Law Journal* (1955), 18:271. This article was also published in the *Journal of the American Medical Association* (1955), 159:487-92.

[41] Louisell, in *Ethics in Medical Progress*, pp. 89-90.

A modification of the conventional approach to the disposition of cadavers was advocated by David Daube in a speech at Duke University on December 3, 1969. Instead of locating permission in formal consent, Daube proposed that the use of dead bodies be restricted *only* by formal objection. Thus, cadavers would ordinarily be available for experimental or teaching or therapeutic (for example, organ donors) purposes *unless* objection was formally lodged (1) by the decedent before death, (2) by the decedent's immediate next-of-kin, or (3) by considerations for justice as, for example, when the body might be required as evidence by a court of law. In the absence of all these objections, Daube's proposal would presume that the dead body is free to serve the living in ways acceptable to current medicine, law, and ethics.

Sir Gerald Nabarro recently introduced two bills into the British Parliament (neither of which passed the Commons) which would have implemented the therapeutic aspect of Daube's proposal. With particular regard for renal transplantation, Sir Gerald's bills would have (1) permitted removal of organs from dead bodies unless the deceased, by explicit instruction, had "contracted-out" during his lifetime, and (2) required establishment of a central renal registry where objections would be recorded.

On balance, the proposals by both Daube and Nabarro have much to commend them; at least they deserve the serious consideration of all those who somehow want to argue that regard for the dead should not hinder the saving of human life. No one to my knowledge (except for Sir Gerald!) has actively supported or advocated legislation of this sort in the West; I am told, however, that such laws are already in force in some northern European countries. The prohibitions in Western culture against mutilation of a corpse have been formulated not so much because of harm done to the dead (of which, obviously, there is none) but because of offense given to the living. It may be that this sentiment largely accounts for repugnance at and resistance to such proposals as these. On the other hand, it does not appear that either proposal does violence to traditional or contemporary principles affecting the disposition of corpses; both proposals merely relocate the initiating responsibility for determining what shall become of one's body after death.

By the phrase "twilight zone," Louisell refers to the present un-certainties about when death occurs. Conventional criteria are compromised by the availability and employment of sophisticated instruments and machines which, in some cases, can artificially maintain a patient's "life" almost indefinitely. This fact, coupled with the need for "fresh" organs in transplantation operations, raises urgent questions about *when* it is permissible to carry out certain procedures ordinarily restricted to dead bodies. We will return to these questions in the next chapter. Meantime, one shares Louisell's opinion that the law is not equipped to give a definitive answer and that considerably more precise reflection and collaborative effort is required among doctors, lawyers, theo-logians, philosophers, and others before an informed consensus can be achieved.[42]

V

The moral issues of human organ transplantation typically oc-cur in the convergence of (1) certain values which we hold with respect to human life and (2) the emergence of innovative medi-cal and surgical techniques which challenge either implicitly or explicitly established precedents and protocols. In practice, this means that values, like statutes, are always in process of being re-formed and that new practices and policies are usually undertaken with restraint until come coherence is established between creed and deed.

Before comparatively recent times, as we have seen, it was not technically feasible to graft human tissues, and the literature of Christian ethics and moral theology has therefore generally not considered whether a healthy person may permit himself to be directly mutilated for the good of a diseased neighbor or the other major moral questions pertaining to human homotransplantation. One could argue, of course, that certain pronouncements and teachings *imply* a Christian response to questions of this sort; but what is taken as implied for one situation may be problem-

[42] *Ibid.*, pp. 91-93.

atical in view of another situation, and erroneous or in need of reformulation.

When Pius XI delivered his famous encyclical on Christian marriage (*Casti Connubii*) in 1930, experiments with human skin grafts had already begun but human organ transplantation was two decades away. Commenting specifically on marriage and the function of human reproductive organs, Pius XI stated:

Christian doctrine establishes, and the light of human reason makes it most clear, that private individuals have no other power over the members of their bodies than that which pertains to their natural ends; and *they are not free to destroy or mutilate their members, or in any other way render themselves unfit for their natural functions, except when no other provision can be made for the good of the whole body.*[43]

Pius XI's reference was particularly to sterilization (and generally to all contraceptive means) in the light of the ancient principle of totality. This principle, as defined by Pius XII in 1952,

asserts that the part exists for the whole and that, consequently, the good of the part remains subordinated to the good of the whole, that *the whole is the determining factor for the part and can dispose of it in its own interests.* . . . The principle of totality itself affirms only this: where the relationship of a whole to its part holds good, and in the exact measure it holds good, *the part is subordinated to the whole and the whole, in its own interests, can dispose of the part.*[44]

Thus the morality of bodily mutilation has been traditionally calculated by Catholic moralists with reference to its necessity "for the health of the whole body or for the preservation of life"[45] of the person mutilated. The moral gravity of the procedure focuses on the question of bodily integrity as defined by the principle of totality, and is calculated in terms of proportionality for the good of the whole body.

[43] Pius XI, "Encyclical on Christian Marriage," (Washington: National Catholic Welfare Conference, 1931), p. 24. Italics added.
[44] Pius XII, "The Moral Limits of Medical Research and Treatment," an Address to the First International Congress on the Histopathology of the Nervous System, *Acta Apostolicae Sedis* (1952), 44:779 ff. Italics added.
[45] Kenny, *Principles of Medical Ethics*, p. 105.

There are occasions, as we have seen,[46] when an action otherwise absolutely prohibited by Catholic teaching, such as abortion or sterilization, may be justified by the rule of double-effect. But this rule, like the principle of totality, refers throughout to the subject undergoing mutilation, and justifies the procedure wholly in terms of its effect upon that same subject. Thus, for example, both sterilization and abortion may be performed in a case of malignant ovarian tumor because (1) the primary intention—to save life—is good, (2) the sterilizing and aborting actions are calculably indirect and unintended, and (3) the operations are undertaken for no other purpose than "for the health of the whole body or for the preservation of life." [47] Neither abortion nor sterilization is licit, however, for other indirect reasons (for example, to safeguard the health or wholeness of the family); and neither is permitted as a direct aggression against nascent life on the grounds that no person has the right to infringe the physical integrity of any other person.

If these traditional principles and their apparent implications were rigorously applied to organ transplantation, no organ could be removed from one person for the benefit of another person; indeed, no human organ could be removed from the person whose natural organ it is unless necessary to the health or preservation of life of that person. On this view there would be as much moral objection to the transplantation of paired as of unpaired organs in cases where the donor was not held to be the primary beneficiary. That this is a widely held maxim is attested, as we have seen, by the declaratory judgments of the Supreme Judicial Court of Massachusetts, which permitted organ donation by minors on grounds that included the opinion, supported by psychiatric testimony, that the operation was necessary for the continued good health and future well-being of the *donor*. But this, it is arguable, was hardly a legitimate extension of the spirit (and surely not the letter) of the principle at issue. Nevertheless it does demonstrate how inflexible and rigid rules evoke tortured rationalizations in morally ambiguous situations.

[46] Chap. 1, *supra*, p. 31.
[47] Kenny, *Principles of Medical Ethics*, p. 105.

As a *general* rule the principle of totality is cogent and useful; it respects individual personal integrity and places the burden of proof upon those who wish in any way and for whatever purpose to compromise it. It is probably fair to say, moreover, that Protestants as well as Catholics, and doctors and lawyers as well as theologians, immediately grasp the importance of the principle and embrace it *as a general rule.* In view of the viability of human homografting, however, it merits asking whether it is morally permissible for a healthy person to be directly mutilated for the benefit of an unhealthy neighbor. One of the more obvious moral difficulties encountered by human homografting in the light of conventional interpretations of totality is that the principle is wholly egocentric. There can be no serious option for altruism or self-sacrifice when it is assumed that what it means for one to be a whole person is substantively defined by reference to bodily components; an assumption which rests, in turn, upon a certain understanding of the limits within which persons may licitly exercise control over their bodies. Of course, the principle may be rationalized, as it was in the Massachusetts court judgments; but this way of dealing with the primary issues finally begs the question. In the end it is a curious Christian mandate (as well as dubious social philosophy) that decisions affecting one's own body should refer to narrow self-interest as the definitive legitimizing criterion. But perhaps this only reflects one of the profound faults in Western philosophy and theology, and that is the tendency to treat ambiguous alternatives as merely either/or choices. When we are mature enough to acknowledge that there are many factors present in our decision-making, and that particular choices are usually the function of particular ingredients in a particular mix, we will no longer require the fiction of either/or formulations imposed (as it were) from outside ourselves, but celebrate our ambiguous freedom with conscious recognition that even our most altruistic motivations are confused with selfishness, and vice-versa. Bernard Häring, responding to those whose object to any homotransplantation on grounds of mutilation and infringement of right order, has made the point succinctly: "It is surely the mark of the most profound reverence toward one's neighbor to be willing to sacrifice—for serious reasons—an organ of one's own body for him in his necessity." [48]

VI

There is no doubt that personality, as we ordinarily think of it, presupposes embodiment and that our bodies are therefore important as *preconditional* to our being persons. But that is not to say that who we are *as persons* is defined by either primary or exclusive reference to our bodies, or that our personhood does not transcend in important ways the limitations imposed by our bodies. Indeed, in view of the whole ethos of modern knowledge of ourselves and our environment, including our bodies, it is no longer reasonable to think of personhood or mind or body or tissue as static entities; flux and change and growth and decay are the pervasive facts of our existence. Thus, it is not only difficult to specify the *precise* state of body in all its aspects at any given moment; it is similarly problematic to identify in some rigid way what we mean by "self" or "person." Most of us, in fact, operate with a fairly free-wheeling self-understanding: consistent enough to provide a sense of stability, but open to the possibility of erratic and irrational moments as reminders that we are living organisms and not automatons.

In this connection I've sometimes wondered how much of my body I could be without before ceasing to be myself; an arm or leg, or eyes or larynx, or perhaps a kidney, or half my stomach, or something else. Conversely, in contemplating the personal dimension of organ transplantation, I have sometimes wondered how many organs from other persons could be transplanted into my body (presuming immunologic acceptance of them!) before I would no longer be myself. Where, indeed, does one draw the line? It should come as no surprise that these ruminations have not afforded a precise answer! When one appreciates that whoever he is is profoundly wrapped up in an incalculable number of variables, that these are constantly shifting, and that in some measure (however modest) who he is and how he perceives him-

[48] Häring, *The Law of Christ*, III, 242.

self is changing with these changing variables, he discovers that it is humanly beyond his grasp, except in the most general terms, to anticipate quantitative losses or additions that would in turn, metamorphose that irreducible quality which is one's self. Making new friends or reading a book or living for a time in a strange culture may affect personality in ways not fundamentally unlike the loss or addition of part of one's body. The difference, in fact, may be more appearance than reality.

Herman Kahn has told the bizarre (and, to date, apocryphal!) story of a commuter train wreck which more or less seriously injured one hundred men. Surgeons called to the spot were able to reconstruct thirty men from the spare parts of the tangled bodies; and afterward, the wives of the original hundred were told, "Now you can fight over them!" Certainly it is an outrageous story, and some would say that it is patently absurd; but it is not wholly unthinkable, and the nervous twitter usually evoked by its telling is evidence of our profound discomfort with some of the hard choices being forced upon us by modern biological science and medical technology. Where to draw the line is far from clear.

At the very least, I think it arguable that who one is most fundamentally is a *person-in-relationships* and that any action which destroys or denigrates the capacity for meaningful relationships is therefore destructive of selfhood or *humanum* as we know it. This is a principle no less applicable to biological science and medical technology than it is to housing, education, employment, and all those other humanizing influences which we regard as indispensable to personal development and maturation. Relationships themselves may be altered, of course, and in that case we may simply become a more or less different self, perceiving and intending ourselves and the world in ways that are more or less different from former ways. But to deny or deprive a human being of the capacity and opportunity for meaningful relationships, both with himself and others, so far jeopardizes our understanding of words like "self" and "person" as to render them meaningless in common discourse.[49] For to be a human person is not a matter

[49] For a sensitive assessment of the responsibility of investigators, with special reference to experiments in isolation and sensory deprivation involving

of *statically* being a certain kind of substance, but a matter of *becoming* personal through temporal duration. And this means that personal being and becoming is a matter of *variable degree* which is referable to one's being more or less fully and intensely personal. That, I suspect, is why old friends are more fully personal than new acquaintances and why members of one's immediate family are dearer than old friends. Personal life is achieved not merely by becoming and living as an individual self but also by becoming and living in interpersonal relationships, because personal maturity occurs only within the context of such personalizing relationships.

The relational context does not rigidly determine the personal development of the individual by shaping him to some predetermined mold, but it does provide a network, a relational field, within which personal becoming and living is evoked from the developing individual. Now there is nothing strange or sinister about this, as those of us who perceive and intend ourselves and the world as Christians ought to know. Indeed, it would not be impious to say in this context that nowhere does incarnational theology speak more clearly and relevantly and profoundly to the humanization of life: the precondition of human selfhood is God's gift of himself in a personal way. Jesus is the possibility of our authentic humanity because we can humanly respond and relate to him. It is thus an article of Christian faith that our lives realize their authentic human possibility in the measure to which we freely and obediently respond to God in Christ. It can be said a number of ways; but the sum of it is that being and becoming a human person means entering into personalizing relationships; and not transgressing a person's capacity or opportunity to do that indicates where we can begin, however tentatively and provisionally, to draw a line between what we will and will not do in regard to ourselves and our bodies.[50]

---

human subjects, see Bernard Bressler, Albert J. Silverman, Sanford I. Cohen, and Barry Shmavonian, "Research in Human Subjects and the Artificial Traumatic Neurosis: Where Does Our Responsibility Lie?" *American Journal of Psychiatry* (1959), 116:522-26.

[50] I prefer to say "will and will not" rather than "can and can not" or "may and may not" because the choice, I think, is still ours to make. The bedrock question which confronts us is whether we will opt for the morally

The dilemma we face, as Professor Samuel Stumpf has pointed out, is "how to achieve two highly desirable goals, namely, the expansion of medical knowledge and the protection of the dignity and the security of the individual." [51] These goals, as Stumpf makes clear, are far from being mutually exclusive; in fact, each is a co-implicate of the other, and especially in clinical situations where human beings are used as experimental subjects. The momentum gained by the discovery of one bit of knowledge impels the investigator to take the next logical step toward gaining further knowledge, and this in turn requires pushing back the moral boundaries which have, to this point, limited research of a given sort.[52] It does not follow, of course, that since these goals are not necessarily mutually exclusive, and that since they in some degree co-implicate each other, that they always may be harmonized; indeed, sometimes they cannot be. Nevertheless, together with whatever other reasons might be put forward in support of an ethics which is tentative without being expedient and provisional without being extempore, this is a persuasive pragmatic justification for resisting rigid and static rules of conduct. New occasions do teach new duties, yesterday's extraordinary measures are today's ordinary procedures, and today's daring experiments often become tomorrow's accepted therapy. Specific acts may therefore vary from time to time and situation to situation in terms of their moral desirability or social acceptance or technical feasibility. Similarly, what we understand to be the value and dignity of a human being is subject to altered meanings in different ages and contexts. But what is constant (not to say static) and coherent (not to say consistent) amid pervasive change and flux is the principal value of human personality which both the means and ends of expanding medical knowledge must serve. On this point I think there is no serious disagreement in Western culture.

---

desirable, the technologically feasible, or the socially permitted; or, more accurately, which combination of these and in what relative proportion?

[51] Samuel E. Stumpf, "Momentum and Morality in Medicine," *The Changing Mores of Biomedical Research*, ed. J. R. Elkinton (*Annals of Internal Medicine*, Vol. 67, No. 3, Part II, Supplement 7, September, 1967), p. 11.

[52] *Ibid.*, pp. 12-13.

In one sense, of course, all medicine and surgery is experimental; but it is not at this general level that the issues of human experimentation commonly emerge. The occasions which give rise to concern for the value and dignity of human persons are those in which what the physician-investigator does is primarily not for the sake of the patient's health and well-being but for the purpose of gaining and extending scientific information. Professor Irving Ladimer has put the point clearly:

Properly conducted experimentation [in man] by qualified scientists must . . . be considered an integral branch of biologic and medical science, but it does not thereby become customary medical practice. Nor does its essentiality and acceptance establish clearly its character or place the methods employed beyond scrutiny. The responsible professions have a duty to delineate for their own members and for a critically vigilant public the nature of medical research and the limits within which it may be properly undertaken.[53]

This view is reflected within the medical profession itself. Dr. Henry Beecher has written that

every act of a doctor designed soundly to relieve or cure a given patient is experimentation of an easily justifiable kind. The patient's placement of himself in the doctor's hands is evidence of consent. The problem becomes a knotty one when the acts of the physician are directed not toward benefit of the patient present but toward patients in general. Such action requires the explicit consent of the *informed* patient. It also requires more than this: it requires profound thought and consideration on the part of the physician, for the complexities of medicine are in some cases so great, it is not reasonable to expect that the patient can be adequately informed as to the full implications of what his consent means.[54]

It is of more than passing interest that doctors themselves have typically been in the front ranks in criticizing experiments which involve human subjects, and this fact itself gives strong support to the argument that the most effective policing of professional conduct can best be done by the profession itself. There are, never-

[53] Irving Ladimer, "Human Experimentation: Medico-Legal Aspects," *New England Journal of Medicine* (1957), 257:18-24.
[54] Henry K. Beecher, *Experimentation in Man* (Springfield, Illinois: Charles C. Thomas, n. d.), p. 43.

theless, a number of quasi-legal and quasi-public bodies in the United States, in addition to national and international codifications by medical groups,[55] which formulate and review policies and procedures within research institutions themselves. In a perceptive and thorough article, Professor John Fletcher has demonstrated that the most important of these originate within the federal government and its health agencies.[56] Despite obvious political implications, it is arguable that these bodies constitute an extension of the principle of intraprofessional self-discipline, a situation which may be all the more significant in view of the fact that there are no judicial decisions which have "considered research specifically in terms of the right and liability of a trained professional to use a living patient or a normal subject as a means of discovering new knowledge not necessarily of direct benefit to that patient or subject." [57]

In the absence of judicial precedent, responsibility for alleged breaches in experimental protocols has largely devolved upon the quasi-legal and quasi-public bodies. One of the most important procedural instances of this kind occurred in the 1966 censure of Drs. Chester Southam and Emanuel Mandel by the Regents of the University of the State of New York. These physicians had injected live cancer cells into twenty-two patients at the Jewish Chronic Disease Hospital in order to test the immune-response mechanism in the seriously ill. Charges were brought against them, not because of the experiment, but because they had failed to inform the patients of the particular kind of cells to be injected. Specifically, they were accused of having obtained consent fraudulently. In due course, the physicians were found guilty and their licenses suspended for one year, but the sentence was stayed on

[55] A selection of "Certain Codes, Declarations, and Recommendations Concerning Medical Ethics and Human Experimentation" is contained in *The Changing Mores of Biomedical Research*, pp. 72-77.

[56] John Fletcher, "Human Experimentation: Ethics in the Consent Situation," in Clark C. Havighurst, ed., *Medical Progress and the Law* (*Law and Contemporary Problems*, Vol. 32, No. 4, Autumn, 1967), pp. 621 ff.

[57] *Ibid.*, p. 623, quoting S. M. Sessoms, "What Hospitals Should Know About Investigational Drugs—Guiding Principles in Medical Research Involving Humans," *Hospitals, Journal of the American Hospital Association* (1958), 32:44.

condition of their good behavior.[58] Fletcher observed that the Regents' decision is of legal significance "because it was made by a legislatively appointed body and could possibly be persuasive to a court deciding a case involving similar circumstances. Of perhaps deeper significance is the vast effect that this widely publicized decision had in deepening public awareness of medical research in humans and of the central importance of informed consent." [59]

Dr. Delford Stickel, a surgeon with considerable experience in renal homografting, has delineated the decision-making process— as it bears upon medical treatment, education, and research and the value of human life—with reference to three parties in the clinical setting: (1) the physician in charge of a patient or research project, (2) a reviewing authority, and (3) the patient himself.[60] He has argued that respect for all three parties not only honors their individual integrity but also gives most promise of protecting their respective interests. This may be no more than a surgeon's good common sense, but there are not many other ways to state the interdependence of idealism and pragmatism so succinctly.

It is generally recognized, and particularly by doctors, that informed and voluntary consent can be a very elusive commodity indeed. Given the complexities of experimental medicine and surgery it is often unreasonable to expect, as Beecher states, that a patient will always be fully informed; and it then becomes a matter of professional judgment whether a given subject is *adequately* informed. Similarly, given the full range of subtle constraints which affect all of us, no decision is *wholly* voluntary in the sense that coercion in some form is entirely absent in the moment of choosing; and it then becomes again a matter of critical assessment whether a given subject has been encouraged and permitted to optimize his limited freedom.

[58] The text of the Regents' decision in the Southam-Mandel case is reprinted in a discussion of the action by Elinor Langer, "Human Experimentation: New York Verdict Affirms Patients' Rights," *Science*, (1966), 151: 6663 ff.

[59] Fletcher, in *Medical Progress and the Law*, p. 624.

[60] Stickel, *Ethics and Moral Aspects of Transplantation*, pp. 275-83.

In addition to these considerations, however, the surest safeguard against abuse in experiments which involve human subjects is the presence of an intelligent, compassionate, and responsible investigator. In one sense, and without diminishing the principal value of human subjects, the investigator in his character and conduct is the key person: it is his responsibility to undertake scientifically significant work, to inform his subjects adequately, and to guarantee the optimal exercise of his subjects' freedom. Such an approach as this removes a number of persons from candidacy for experimental subjects; among them minors, prisoners, the terminally ill, and mental defectives. A final protection against irresponsibility in human experimentation was recently put forward by Dr. M. H. Pappworth: "No experiment should be contemplated, proposed, or undertaken to which, if he were in circumstances identical to those of the intended subjects, the experimenter would even hesitate to submit himself, or members of his own family, or anybody for whom he had any respect or affection." [61]

Despite Pappworth's location of the baseline reference for justification of action in self-interest, what he has proposed is one way of deriving a particular application from the Golden Rule and the general Christian obligation to show love. It is not the only way, to be sure, and some would doubtless argue that it is not the best way. The difficulty we typically encounter in the relationship between Christian love and social (i.e., interpersonal) action is that the former often seems to be too vague when confronted by a particular problematic and the latter too restricted in its viable alternatives when faced with the general obligation to love.

One way to deal with that difficulty, without establishing a legalistic correspondence between love and any particular action or leaving the relationship entirely unstructured and open-ended, is expressed in the words "middle axioms." John Bennett, following the original suggestion of W. A. Visser 't Hooft and J. H. Oldham,[62] defines a "middle axiom" as "more concrete than a universal ethical principle and less specific than a program that

[61] M. H. Pappworth, *Human Guinea Pigs—Experimentation on Man* (London: Routledge & Kegan Paul, 1967), p. 189.
[62] Cf. W. A. Visser 't Hooft and J. H. Oldham, *The Church and Its Function in Society* (London: G. Allen & Unwin, 1937), p. 210.

includes legislation and political strategy." [63] An example of this approach to decision-making can be found in the writings of physicians themselves, illustrative of which is the following collation of moral guidelines suggested by Drs. J. R. Elkinton and Eugene D. Robin:[64]

1. Compassionate concern for the patient as a total person is the primary goal of the physician and the investigator.
2. Organ transplantation should have some reasonable possibility of clinical success.
3. The transplant must be undertaken only with an acceptable therapeutic goal as its purpose.
4. Risk to the healthy donor of an organ must be kept low, but such risk should not be a contra-indication to the voluntary offer of an organ by an informed donor.
5. There must be complete honesty with the patient and his family, including every benefit of available general medical knowledge and of specific information concerning transplantation.
6. Each transplantation should be conducted under a protocol which ensures the maximum possible addition to scientific knowledge.
7. Careful, intensive, and objective evaluation of results of independent observers is mandatory.
8. A careful, accurate, conservative approach to the dissemination of information to public news media is desirable.

In the present situation and on the assumption that transplantation of paired organs will continue to require living donors for whom there are calculable health risks—these axioms represent an interdisciplinary moral consensus which draws upon and incorporates value postulates from law, medicine, and theology alike. There are those, of course, who challenge the assumption that living donors should continue to be used for human homografting; the moral ambiguities attendant upon using living

---

[63] John C. Bennett, *Christian Ethics and Social Policy* (New York: Charles Scribner's Sons, 1946), p. 77.

[64] Cf. Elkinton, "Moral Problems in the Use of Borrowed Organs, Artificial and Transplanted," p. 363; and Robin, "Rapid Scientific Advances," pp. 624-5.

donors, together with the clinical risks and uncertainties, are held to be so great that scientific and technical effort should be refocused largely, if not entirely, upon developing mechanical and/ or cadaveric resources, with a view toward eventual abandonment of living donors as a source of organ supply. The sentiment expressed in this demurrer is doubtless agreeable in principle to most (if not all) of us, inasmuch as it is true that the use of protheses or cadaveric organs would plainly obviate present concerns in regard to living donors. *In the present situation,* however, we simply do not have these options before us as immediate operational alternatives, and, therefore, guidelines for the use of living donors—until the time that other options are functionally available—are both useful and imperative.

Moreover, as we have argued, the morality of using living donors—even in the present stage of homografting with its attendant scientific and technical risks and limitations—is not wholly defined by the apparent necessity for human organs. The principal moral question is still whether a healthy person may licitly permit himself to be mutilated for the good of a diseased neighbor. If that question be answered affirmatively—as I think it should be, within certain limits—all that remains is to structure procedural protocols which guarantee and protect the humane interests of the parties concerned. Sacrificial love, on occasion, may permit—and even oblige—one to lay down his life for his friend; in the case of organ transplantation, love for a neighbor can similarly allow—and even constrain—one to sacrifice his own organ for his friend in his distress.

IV

Death and Care of the Dying

A commonly accepted principle among us, and one particularly emphasized in medical education, is that the mission and duty of doctors and nurses is to prolong life and relieve suffering. The corollary doctrine, as I have often heard it from doctors themselves, is that death is the enemy.[1] And when the positive means for implementing these principles are exhausted, it is usual to enjoin the counterprinciple: do no harm.

At the time that these maxims were first formulated, relatively clear and valid distinctions were doubtless signified; but it is becoming increasingly apparent in our time that those ancient distinctions are blurred by advances in biomedical technology, surgical skill, and chemotherapy. It sometimes happens nowadays that preserving life and relieving pain are not two sides of the same coin which neatly complement each other; instead they present themselves as alternative courses of action which are often in conflict and occasionally mutually exclusive. Sometimes life can be extended only by the accompaniment of great pain and personal sacrifice as, for example, in cases of spina bifida; sometimes distress and agony can be relieved only at the eventual expense of life itself as, for example, in the administration of pain-

---

[1] There is, of course, biblical precedent for this attitude—if one reads Paul *out of context*. Cf. I Corinthians 15:26.

relieving drugs to toxic dosages. With increasing frequency, where to draw the line between prolonging life and relieving pain is an uncertain point.

Moreover, there was a time, certainly in contrast with our own time, when the scientific criteria for pronouncing death were relatively simple and when the technological means available for interfering with death were relatively limited. But that time, also, is no more. Formerly, it could be generally agreed that death occurred when vital life processes stopped; now, however, those same processes can often be indefinitely maintained or prolonged by mechanical or surgical or pharmacologic assistance. Formerly, human life was understood to be coterminous with "natural" vitality; now, however, it has become possible to maintain natural bodily functions long after the human organism has ceased to be intentionally, self-directingly, and purposively viable. In view of wide-ranging advances in both the arts and the sciences, a dramatic and urgent modern question is what we now mean when we speak of life and death that are distinctively human and personal.

These and cognate questions, as I have argued earlier, are matters of concern not only to the medical profession but to all who venture to address themselves to humane interests. Innovations in medicine and surgery constitute only some—albeit often the most dramatic—of the alterations in modern life which give rise to these problems. Concern for guaranteed levels of family income, decent housing, adequate education, sufficient nutrition, effective political participation, and all the other social and cultural opportunities we think important, expresses (though sometimes only inchoately) the perception of modern man that more than organismic vitality is at stake when we speak of persons or human beings and the ways they are to be treated. To be sure, bodily health and vitality are *preconditional* to being a human person in this larger sense, and we are therefore appropriately concerned for physical well-being. But the difference between our time and former times may well be that life-vitality and human well-being can no longer be accepted as coterminous or synonymous categories. Persons need healthy bodies, and nobody seriously challenges that point, but they require more than healthy bodies if they are to be persons in any authentic and currently meaningful sense of that word.

Some of our primitive ancestors observed that a man grows steadily weaker as he loses blood; and they concluded, quite logically but erroneously, that a man's life—all his experience, strengths, and characteristics—is therefore contained in his blood.[2] Following such reasoning, Pliny's *Natural History* recommended that epileptics might benefit from quaffing the fresh, warm blood of a gladiator not yet dead! Modern science has not altered the basic observation—a man does grow steadily weaker as he loses blood; but the conclusion has been radically changed and stripped of magic and superstition. Blood is preconditional to life, but man does not live by blood alone! More to the point, if what we conventionally mean by human life is no more than biologic vitality, I would argue that man does not live by life alone. It is no abuse of the gospel to paraphrase Jesus in this way; and neither is it inconsistent with his proclamation that a man's life does not consist in his possessions, that we require more than bread for life, and that the "abundant life" does not denigrate but nevertheless transcends mere physical existence.

That Western culture is *de facto* Judeo-Christian in its orientation, irrespective of the particular ways in which individuals and groups formulate their beliefs and values, means that we cannot divorce a particular religious and philosophical tradition from the ways in which we undertake to resolve the particular problems of professional ethics. Somewhere, somehow, however, we have succumbed to the temptation to seek and affirm the lowest common natural denominator as definitive of life (namely, vitality); and now, in the wake of scientific and technological advance that bids fair to outstrip our moral imagination and sensitivity and confuse all the old simplifications, we are hard-pressed to say with any assurance of purpose who we are, where we are going, and how we can coordinate means and ends.

It is appropriate, therefore, that some of our cherished presuppositions be reexamined and that some of our uncritically

---

[2] The interdependency of life and blood is noted in a number of biblical passages, among them Deuteronomy 12:23, "the blood is the life," and Leviticus 17:14, "the life of all flesh is the blood thereof."

accepted assumptions be tested with reference to current problematics. Among these is the notion that the doctor's primary mission is to prolong life. If it is true, as I think it is, that life (in the sense of functioning organ systems) is preconditional to human health and well-being, the force of that proposition is in turn authenticated by the converse assertion that health and well-being, or at least the promise of them, are preconditional to life in any humanly meaningful sense. The Hippocratic Oath itself emphasizes that the *summum bonum* is not merely biological life but the patient's well-being. Practical circumstances make us increasingly aware that life and well-being are not always complementary and, to that extent, support the ancient wisdom of the Oath. Perhaps it is no more than professional *hubris*—the doctor's pride and personal sense of well-being that come from conquering disease and death—that has encouraged and accepted the correspondence of life and well-being. Whatever the reasons, the notion that biologic vitality is the highest good deserves serious and sober examination.

In addition to examining the value theory of the Hippocratic Oath, we may note that our popular as well as professional tendency to regard death as a wholly negative value is a questionable, if not aberrant, attitude when viewed within the perspective of Judeo-Christian faith. No one can seriously doubt that theologians and pastors, together with doctors and lawyers, share large responsibility for the view that death is the enemy, a bad thing, and to be avoided or overcome at (almost!) whatever cost. Still, and despite the paradox, we must probably look to these disciplines more than to any other for a fitting and responsible understanding of this experience for which all of us are destined but of which none of us has better than secondhand and vicarious knowledge.

I

Until comparatively recent times, questions about when a person died and what criteria certified death were thought to be settled. Indeed, some medical textbooks of not very long ago were still commending the use of a mirror or feather to detect exhala-

tion; and the entire matter of deciding whether death had occurred was treated as a simple and straightforward judgment
which could be reliably made on the basis of certain unambiguous
signs. These signs were typically the cessation or absence of spontaneous life; and by that was meant the cessation or absence of
sensibility, respiration, and circulation.

Judicial definitions of the death of persons thus commonly
referred to "departure from life," [3] "the cessation of his physical
life," [4] or, more specifically, "a total stoppage of the circulation of
the blood and cessation of the animal and vital functions consequent thereon, such as respiration, pulsation, etc." [5] More recently, and probably in order to take into account new techniques and
sophisticated instrumentation for resuscitation, low temperature
cooling, and heart-lung support, a decision by the Kansas Supreme
Court broadened judicial interpretation of the criteria for defining
death to include "the complete cessation of all vital functions
without possibility of resuscitation." [6]

In view of the wide-ranging diversity and dissimilarity in definitions of death, Professors Martin Halley and William Harvey of
the Washburn University School of Law in Topeka have argued
the need for a definition "as unambiguous and exact as possible"
which will be acceptable and functional for both lawyers and
doctors. Because the law operates best when data are objective
and precise, Halley and Harvey insist that definitions of "functional death"—sometimes employed when supportive instrumentation maintains vital life processes after total and irreversible
destruction of the central nervous system—are too indefinite and
diverse and that nothing less than irreversible cessation of *all* the
vital organ systems (cerebral, respiratory, and circulatory) will
suffice as definitive of the moment of a person's death. In order to
demonstrate that medicine and law are close to general agreement,

[3] *Finch* v. *Edwards,* 239 Mo. App. 788, 198 S. W. (2d) 665, 670 (1947).
[4] American Law Institute, *Restatement of the Law of Property* (St. Paul:
American Institute Publishers, 1940), p. 1325.
[5] *Thomas* v. *Anderson,* 96 Cal. App. (2d) 371, 215 P. (2d) 478 (1950).
[6] *United Trust Company* v. *Pyke,* 199 Kan. 1, 4, 427 P. (2d) 67, 71
(1967). Italics added.

the components of their respective definitions of death were juxtaposed as follows:

Components of Definitions of Death

Commonly Accepted but Unofficial Medical Definition	Evolving but Unofficial Legal Definition
1. Insensibility	1. Cessation of "vital functions"
2. Cessation of respiration	2. Cessation of respiration
3. Cessation of circulation	3. Cessation of circulation
4. Irreversibility	4. Impossibility of resuscitation

On the basis of this apparent compatibility, Halley and Harvey proposed that death be defined, for both medicine and law, as "irreversible cessation of *all* of the following: (1) total cerebral function, (2) spontaneous function of the respiratory system, and (3) spontaneous function of the circulatory system." [7]

On the face of it, there seems to be enough uniformity among the various components to warrant such a definition. Closer examination, however, shows that agreement between these professions is not so self-evident. The editor of the *Journal of the American Medical Association*, in response to the Halley-Harvey article, commented on the difficulty of assigning *objective* meaning to the component combinations of (1) insensibility—cessation of vital functions and (4) irreversibility—impossibility of resuscitation. These, he said,

give the most trouble, not because they differ in meaning (which they do not) or in wording (which they do), but because both embody an element of judgment and prognostication without offering any objective measure of final dissolution. . . . When all is said and done, it seems ironic that the end point of existence, which ought to be as clear and sharp as in a chemical titration, should so defy the power

[7] M. Martin Halley and William F. Harvey, "Medical vs. Legal Definitions of Death," *Journal of the American Medical Association* (1968), 204:423-25.

of words to describe it and the power of men to say with certainty, "It is here." [8]

Beyond this caveat by the *Journal of the American Medical Association's* editor, I would want to add that any definition which treats death only or chiefly as a *biological event* rather than a *personal process* will encounter the most serious practical and theoretical difficulties, not only from the biological sciences but from theology and philosophy as well. Both these dimensions are more or less present in every instance of human death and both deserve consideration in any serious attempt to get behind the elaborate mythology that protects us from the reality of death. That we have tended to emphasize the *impersonal* and *objective* aspects of a biological event over which, for one or another reason, we ourselves exercise little or no control has presumably made death—at least for those who stand by and watch it happen—less painful and anxiety-producing. But this, as anyone who has realistically faced his own death knows, is an elegant dodge, a fantasy, a dishonesty; and it is all these things and more, for what it does to one's own perception of himself and his death as well as for what it does to deprive another person in the process of his dying of the dignity and meaning due himself and his own death.

Dr. John B. Graham, a professor of pathology and also a perceptive observer of professional mores, has written that physicians are no more immune to the anxieties of death than other Americans; nor are they less fearful of the existential reality of death, or less determined to expunge the word and thought of this reality from vocabulary and experience. "Most Americans, including physicians," says Dr. Graham, "are not living authentically, because we are afraid to face up to ultimate issues." Illustrative of this tendency are the kinds of answers typically given to a question like, "What does it mean to die?" According to Dr. Graham, "this might be answered with a description of the phenomenon as observed with respect to civilization, nations, persons, cells, even molecules, plus a complex discussion of the relation of the nitrogen-carbon cycle to immortality. But this would be a smoke

[8] Editorial, "What and When Is Death?" *Journal of the American Medical Association* (1968), 204:540.

screen." [9] And so it would, for such descriptions would tend to objectify dying by precise measurement when, in fact, these objective considerations are preconditional to, but not definitive of, the process.

II

It is generally well known that brain cells are especially sensitive to anoxia; the cerebral cortical cells begin to die within five minutes of arrested circulation of oxygenated blood, and the whole brain is usually considered dead after fifteen minutes. Other systems and organs deteriorate more slowly: the heart can be stimulated to spontaneous activity after several minutes of inaction; kidneys can still function after as much as an hour following nephrectomy; muscle can survive for several hours; and corneal transplants can be successfully performed days after surgical removal. Dr. Pierre H. Muller of Lille has suggested that "agonochemistry" (the study of "chemical changes immediately preceding death, and half way between biochemistry and thanatochemistry"), together with research in cellular mechanisms, will one day "produce a pathognomonic biological or pathological test the clinicians are looking for to diagnose death when the tissues are being maintained artificially." Thus, Muller thinks it deserves emphasizing that "death is a process and not a moment in time as the law believes." [10]

Dr. H. P. Wasserman of South Africa agrees that death is a biological process, but argues that there are many kinds of death and that each of these deserves special consideration: "Cytological death, organ death, spiritual death, theological death, legal death, social death, physiological death and pathological death are terms which denote specialized interest in the life or cessation of life in an individual. We must therefore define life and death in an *individual* and not in any of its component parts." [11] "The Dec-

[9] John B. Graham, "Acceptance of Death—Beginning of Life," *North Carolina Medical Journal* (1963), 24:319, 317.

[10] Pierre H. Muller, "Legal Medicine and the Delimitation of Death," *World Medical Journal* (1967), 14: 142, 140.

[11] H. P. Wasserman, "Problematical Aspects of the Phenomenon of

laration of Sydney," a statement on death unanimously adopted by the World Medical Association in 1968, echoed a similar opinion when it noted "that clinical interest lies not in the state of preservation of isolated cells, but in the fate of the person, and that the time of death of various body cells and organs is less important than the determination that the process has become irreversible, irrespective of resuscitation techniques that may be employed." [12]

In view of the fact that death, however conceived, is not an identical or even uniform human experience—an observation which is as valid biologically and neurophysiologically as it is theologically and philosophically—these points are well taken. We surely cannot diminish the biological aspects of death; but neither can they be determinative of what we mean when we speak of the death of a human being. In the long run it would probably serve us better to understand the relationship between biological vitality and death in much the same way we perceive the relationship between biological vitality and life: the cessation of spontaneous function in *all* the great organ systems may be preconditional for death but not definitive or determinative of it. If we want to attach significance to human death, clearly differentiated from the significance we attach to plant or animal death, the human factor which denominates that significance must somehow be articulated in terms that are especially appropriate to it and not to all the rest of creation as well. It was this aspect of the matter which Professor Gunnar Biörk of Stockholm had in mind when he wrote that "when considering the definition of death it seems essential to separate the problem of the *concept* of death from that of the *procedure* in stating and pronouncing death on the basis of any one concept." [13]

At this point it is worth remembering that the urgency of the

Death," *World Medical Journal* (1967), 14:147. For a similar opinion, expressed by an American physician, cf. Henry K. Beecher, "Scarce Resources and Medical Advancement," *Daedalus* (1969), 98:291.

[12] "Moment of Death," *British Medical Association News* (October, 1968), 13:1.

[13] Gunnar Biörk, "On the Definition of Death," *World Medical Journal* (1967), 14:138.

modern question has been largely propelled into public and professional prominence by two related developments in biomedical engineering and surgical science: the care of hopelessly and irreversibly unconscious patients and the possibilities generated by organ transplantation. The innovations in these fields put our current problems with death and the management of dying patients into perspective.

Questions having to do with the care of irreversibly unconscious and/or dying patients have an antecedent moral priority because the traditions of Christian faith and Western culture assign certain inalienable rights to persons irrespective of qualifying circumstances. This is the preeminent reason that procedures for carrying out organ transplantations, when the prospective donor is hopelessly unconscious or terminally ill, are formally acknowledged by individual doctors and professional organizations alike to be subordinate to the care of the prospective donor as a patient in his own right. Thus the World Medical Association and many national groups of physicians have agreed to the principle that "if transplantation of an organ is involved [after death], the decision that death exists should be made by two or more physicians and the physicians determining the time of death should in no way be immediately concerned with the performance of the transplantation." [14]

Commenting upon the considerable ethical importance of separating the care of dying patients from the needs of prospective organ recipients, Professor Paul Ramsey has argued that any effort to define more precisely the moment of death should be

so that persons who have died need not have "life"-sustaining measures inflicted upon their unburied corpses, needlessly and at great expense to their families. The reasons for this must be sufficient in themselves as proper medical practice. Any benefit that may accrue to other patients in this age of organ transplantation must be a wholly independent by-product of an updating of death that is already per se right and wise and a proper judgment to be made concerning the primary patient. The issues that have been "simmering" for a long time must be resolved as if transplantation did not exist as a surgical

[14] British Medical Association News (October, 1968). See also The New York Times, August 10, 1968.

therapy. There is sufficient need and sufficient reason, I have suggested, for withholding (in the face of life and without a pronouncement of death) extraordinary measures in caring for the irreversibly dying.[15]

Whether we can in fact discuss death "as if transplantation did not exist" is a possibility about which I have more doubt than Professor Ramsey; but that questions relating to transplantation must be set apart—"bracketed," as phenomenologists would say—from renewed consideration of the criteria and definition of death is indisputable. There are many reasons to commend this approach, some of which have been indicated in the preceding paragraphs. In the end, they all have more or less to do with judging, as best we can, when a person's death is appropriate.

III

Although it is too infrequently a topic of casual conversation or scholarly essays, most of us probably agree that there is a time when it is appropriate for a human being to die. The difficulty with this otherwise generally acceptable maxim lies in trying to say specifically *when* it is fitting that a particular person die. The patient's dilemma has been vividly described by the colleague of a doctor who himself experienced the agony of not being allowed to die:

A doctor aged sixty-eight was admitted to an overseas hospital after a barium meal had shown a large carcinoma of the stomach. He had retired from practice five years earlier, after severe myocardial infarction had left his exercise tolerance considerably reduced. The early symptoms of the carcinoma were mistakenly thought to be due to myocardial ischaemia. By the time the possibility of carcinoma was first considered the disease was already far advanced; laparotomy showed extensive metastatic involvement of the abdominal lymph nodes and liver. Palliative gastrectomy was performed with the object of preventing perforation of the primary tumor into the peritoneal cavity, which appeared to the surgeon to be imminent. Histological examination showed the growth to be an anaplastic primary adenocarcinoma. There was clinical and radiological evidence of secondary deposits in the lower thoracic and lumbar vertebrae.

[15] Ramsey, "On Up-Dating Death," in Donald R. Cutler, ed., *The Religious Situation, 1969* (Boston: Beacon Press, 1969), p. 273.

133

The patient was told of the findings and fully understood their import. In spite of increasingly large doses of pethidine, and of morphine at night, he suffered constantly with severe abdominal pain and pain resulting from compression of spinal nerves by tumor deposits.

On the tenth day after the gastrectomy the patient collapsed with classic manifestations of massive pulmonary embolism. Pulmonary embolectomy was successfully performed in the ward by a registrar. When the patient had recovered sufficiently he expressed his appreciation of the good intentions and skill of his young colleague. At the same time he asked that if he had a further cardiovascular collapse no steps should be taken to prolong his life, for the pain of his cancer was now more than he would needlessly continue to endure. He himself wrote a note to this effect in his case records, and the staff of the hospital knew his feelings.

His wish notwithstanding, when the patient collapsed again, two weeks after the embolectomy—this time with acute myocardial infarction and cardiac arrest—he was revived by the hospital's emergency resuscitation team. His heart stopped on four further occasions during that night and each time was restarted artificially. The body then recovered sufficiently to linger for three more weeks, but in a decerebrate state, punctuated by episodes of projectile vomiting accompanied by generalized convulsions. Intravenous nourishment was carefully combined with blood transfusion and measures necessary to maintain electrolyte and fluid balance. In addition, antibacterial and antifungal antiobiotics were given as prophylaxis against infection, particularly pneumonia complicating the tracheotomy that had been performed to ensure a clear airway. On the last day of his illness, preparations were being made for the work of the failing respiratory centre to be given over to an artificial respirator, but the heart finally stopped before this endeavor could be realized.

This case report is submitted for publication without commentary or conclusions, which are left for those who may read it to provide for themselves.[16]

Most of us probably agree that there *is* an appropriate time to die; the difficulty lies in trying to say with some precision *when* it is fitting for a particular person to die. On rare occasions (capital punishment and war, for example), we as a society are, reluctantly, willing to affirm a more or less specific time for another human being prospectively to die; more often, however, we

[16] W. St. C. Symmers, Sr., "Not Allowed to Die," *British Medical Journal* (1968), 1:442.

find it a good deal easier to say *in retrospect* whether a given individual's death was timely—that is, fitting in his circumstances. Perhaps that is as it should be; at least a cautious and conservative approach to decisions of this sort has, with notable exceptions, protected certain classes of citizens from callous extermination in civilized history. But the question of the appropriate time to die has taken on perplexing and agonizing features in our time, not as a means to rid the body politic of "undersirables" but as a means to ensure a measure of dignity and reverence to those persons who (in our best judgment) are irremediably and fairly immediately faced with the prospect of their own death.

The difficulties currently encountered appear to focus, in the main, on two discrete but interrelated considerations: the *criteria* for determining when death has occurred and a clinical *definition* of death. Both of these are important because there is not only concern for the time of death, as precisely as it can be determined, but also for the time when a doctor pronounces that a given patient has died. These respective times are not always simultaneous. In the end, the time when a physician declares a patient dead may be the more important practical question; but this is not decided without reference to some notion about the time of death *qua* death. Both questions, moreover, bear upon the *meaning* which we attach to death and how we understand and interpret it; and to the extent that this is so, we again cannot exclude philosophy and theology from the discussion.

Whatever else may be said about the time of death, it is now abundantly clear, apart from cases of violent death (as, for example, by a disintegrating explosion), that human death usually occurs as process rather than as a precise moment and that no single criterion is wholly adequate to denote its presence or absence.

On the evening of December 29, 1949, Dr. Hermann N. Sander, a physician in Hillsboro, New Hampshire, was arrested and charged with the murder of Mrs. Abbie C. Borroto, a fifty-nine-year-old cancer patient who had died on December 4.[17] Mrs.

[17] Details of this celebrated case were amply covered in numerous issues of *The New York Times*, December 30, 1949, through March 24, 1950.

Borroto's hospital records attributed death to carcinoma of the large bowel, with metastisis of the liver and inanition (starvation). The state, however, charged that Sander had "feloniously and willfully and of his own malice aforethought killed and murdered" Mrs. Borroto by four intravenous injections of air.

Investigation of the circumstances surrounding Mrs. Borroto's death began when the president of the medical staff at Hillsboro County General Hospital received the monthly report of the record librarian. This report included a notation, dictated and signed by Sander eight days after Mrs. Borroto's death: "Patient was given ten cc. of air intravenously repeated four times. Expired within ten minutes after this was started." At Sander's trial, testimony centered on the question of whether these injections were in fact the cause of death.

Sander had been Mrs. Borroto's physician for one and a half years and had already operated on her for cancer. Following a brief convalescence at home, Mrs. Borroto had returned to the hospital in order to secure more adequate attention and to relieve her husband of the responsibility of attending to her.

Sander testified that Mr. Borroto had constantly pleaded with him to do something about his wife's pain. In her testimony, the record librarian confirmed that the patient had indeed experienced great pain, and that on the day before her death Mrs. Borroto was given several strong doses of drugs (100 to 200 mg. of demarol and pantagon, one-third to one grain at a time) without any obvious effect. Both the husband and a special nurse assigned to Mrs. Borroto corroborated the evidence that drugs were impotent to relieve the patient's pain. Sander further testified that when Borroto stayed up all night on December 3, drinking coffee and worrying about his wife, he (Sander) became concerned about the husband's bad heart.

On the day of Mrs. Borroto's death (December 4) but prior to Sander's administration of the air injections, which he freely admitted doing, the special nurse had found the patient unconscious, her body rigid but convulsed by general spasms, and her extremities cold. Unable to get a pulse, the nurse called Dr. Albert Snay, a member of the hospital staff. Snay was similarly unable to feel a pulse, nor could he detect heartbeat with a stethoscope;

and at the trial he admitted having said at that time that the patient was "practically dead." Immediately after Snay left Mrs. Borroto, Sander entered her room and confirmed Snay's diagnosis by his own examination. He then secured a sterile syringe and injected the air, which he estimated to be only 25-28 cc.

At his trial Sander could give no rational explanation for injecting air into a corpse; he could only say that an "obsession" had come over him and dictated his action, which now made no sense to him. Mrs. Borroto was dead, he said, and on the impulse of "a matter of seconds" he decided to make certain that she experienced no more pain. Notation of the air injections was made in the medical record for no other reason than the doctor's duty to register everything done for a patient.

The autopsy report attributed Mrs. Borroto's death to cancer, starvation, bronchial pneumonia, or a combination of these; and the doctor who performed the autopsy (who was Head of the Department of Legal Medicine at Harvard University) testified that death was not caused by air embolism. More specifically, he stated that blood clots in Mrs. Borroto's brain indicated that her death was gradual and progressive over a period of hours, rather than immediate and momentary. He further stated that, according to experiments, more than 40 cc. of air would be needed to cause the death of a human being.

After deliberating for an hour, Sander's jury (which, incidentally, was composed of nine Roman Catholics and three Protestants) returned a verdict of "not guilty."

There are certain integral aspects of this case which are still discomfiting after all these years. Not least among them is the embarrassing testimony from the two physicians most immediately knowledgeable of the patient's condition at or about the time of her death, one of whom adjudged that she was "practically dead" while the other administered death-dealing injections into what he perceived to be a corpse. Beyond this, there is the manner in which the entire episode came to be investigated. Finally, the opinion of the doctor who performed the autopsy (supported by experiments?) that the amount of air injected was not a lethal dose only adds to the general confusion of testimony.

In view of such conflicting medical evidence, it might seem

reasonable to conclude that the autopsy report was what the jury found convincing. It would be difficult, however, to discount the effect of several tangential factors upon the jury. Among these, the foremost was a petition of support, signed by more than 90 percent of the registered voters in the town, which described Sander as "a man of Christian virtue who has been devoted to the highest interests of human welfare at all times." If one considers the greater weight of the evidence, the motive of mercy probably played a large part in the jury's decision to acquit. And if the full range of testimony, especially that given by the accused and attributed to him, is contemplated, it is not entirely speculative to conclude that Sander's action was largely sponsored by compassion toward his painwracked patient, her anxious husband, and revulsion at his own inability any longer to relieve her distress.

The Sander case remains important, if only because it is one of the very few of its sort—which may be more an occasion for concern than satisfaction. Indeed, according to Professor George P. Fletcher, there has not been a single instance in the annals of Anglo-American judicial proceedings in which (1) a doctor has been convicted of murder or manslaughter for having killed to end the suffering of his patient, or (2) a layman or doctor has been convicted of omitting to take steps that could have averted death.[18] These circumstances may be largely responsible for the fact that, despite Professor Ramsey's proper insistence that questions of death *per se* be separated from considerations of organ transplantation, most of the modern literature discusses the definition and criteria of death with explicit reference to organ transplantation.

IV

Dr. G. P. J. Alexandre, Head of the Department of Renal Transplantation at the University of Louvain, has used nine patients as kidney donors who were victims of severe craniocerebral injury but whose hearts had not stopped.

[18] Cf. George P. Fletcher, "Legal Aspects of the Decision Not to Prolong Life," *Journal of the American Medical Association* (1968), 203:66.

Five conditions were always met in these nine cases: (1) complete bilateral mydriasis [dilation of both pupils]; (2) complete absence of reflexes, both natural and in response to profound pain; (3) complete absence of spontaneous respiration, five minutes after mechanical respiration has been stopped; (4) falling blood pressure, necessitating increasing amounts of vasopressive drugs (either adrenaline or Neosynephrine [phenylephrine hydrochloride]); (5) a flat EEC.[19]

Alexandre was careful to point out that these criteria were employed with reference to a particular type of injury and that all five conditions were met before donor nephrectomy. Thus, in response to the argument that some biologists regard one minute of electroencephalogram silence as incontrovertible proof of death, Alexandre accepted Dr. J. Hamburger's point that a flat EEG can be caused by barbituate poisoning and added that a gas embolism occurring in heart surgery can also produce a flat EEG. More important, he insisted that patients registering a flat EEG as the result of barbituate poisoning or gas embolism would not fulfill the other four conditions, nor would they, in all likelihood, have severe head injuries.

Dr. J. P. Revillard of Lyon has suggested that, in addition to Alexandre's five signs, two other criteria afford even more precise determination of death: "(1) interruption of blood flow in the brain as judged by angiography, which we assume is a better sign of death than a flat EEG, and (2)—of less value—the absence of reaction to atropine." [20]

Not all doctors, however, are satisfied with these criteria, as elaborate and comprehensive as they appear to be. Dr. R. Y. Calne, Professor of Surgery at the University of Cambridge, has stated bluntly that "although Dr. Alexandre's criteria are medically persuasive, according to traditional definitions of death he is in fact removing kidneys from live donors. *I feel that if a patient has a heartbeat he cannot be regarded as a cadaver.*" And Dr. T.E. Starzl, Professor of Surgery at the University of Colorado, echoed the same judgment in speaking of the "living cadaver": "I doubt if any of the members of our transplantation team could accept

[19] G. P. J. Alexandre *et al.*, "Discussion of Murray," in *Ethics in Medical Progress*, p. 69.
[20] *Ibid.*, p. 71.

a person as being dead as long as there was a heartbeat." [21] Further, Dr. G. B. Giertz of Stockholm, arguing against the view that a profoundly comatose patient for whom there is no reasonable chance of recovery should be termed dead even when other vital functions are being mechanically maintained, has insisted that "a person dying is still a person living, and he keeps his elementary human rights up to the moment when life becomes extinct." [22]

In his reply to Giertz, Alexandre stated the crux of the matter and his own assessment of the basic alternatives:

I would like to make it clear that, in my opinion, there has never been and there never will be any question of taking organs from a dying person who has "no reasonable chance of getting better or resuming consciousness." The question is of taking organs from a dead person, and the point is that I *do not accept the cessation of heartbeats as the indication of death.* We are as much concerned with the preservation of life in a dying person as with the preservation of life in a foetus; but I *think irreversible damage to the central nervous system is an indication of physiological death that permits us to take an organ from a body that is already a cadaver.*[23]

The literature on thanatology is increasing with each month's issue of medical, legal, and theological journals. This brief sampling, however, is enough to indicate that among physicians as well as others there is significant diversity of opinion and a good deal of scientific uncertainty and imprecision. At present the discussion seems to fall, as it were, between two stools: the traditional criterion of heart stoppage as synonymous with death and the confusion imparted to that criterion when modern resuscitative and supportive measures are available and employed. When, indeed, is death: when there is massive and irremediable brain damage despite persistent circulation and respiration, or when there is no spontaneous function of the heart despite viable cerebral and respiratory function?

One way into the subtleties and complexities of questions like these is to consider another actual case. In August, 1963, the

[21] *Ibid.,* pp. 73, 70. Italics added.
[22] *Ibid.,* p. 147.
[23] *Ibid.,* pp. 154-55. Italics added.

British Medical Journal reported the case of David Potter:[24]

> A thirty-two-year-old man was admitted to Newcastle General Hospital with multiple skull fractures and extensive brain damage. Fourteen hours after admission, on June 16, he stopped breathing. Artificial respiration was then begun by machine so that one of his kidneys could later be taken for transplantation to another man. After 24 hours of artificial respiration a kidney was taken from the body on June 17. The respirator was then turned off and there was no spontaneous breathing or circulation.

Interest in this case was heightened by the varied comments from the coroner and physicians most closely associated with it. The coroner's opinion was that the patient was alive at the time of nephrectomy, but hopelessly injured, and that the operation was not contributory to death. The attending physician was variously reported as having said (1) that the patient had "virtually died" when he stopped breathing on June 16, but that he had legally died when his heart and circulation stopped on June 17; or (2) that the patient was medically dead on June 16 and legally dead on June 17. A neurologist claimed that brain damage was so extensive and irreparable that the patient was dead before operation, and that mechanical ventilation was employed only in order to allow time for operating preparation. The examining pathologist was satisfied that the cause of death was brain damage and that the nephrectomy did not contribute to death.

Owing to the circumstances of this case, an inquest was held and its findings reported in the *Medico-Legal Journal*:[25]

> An inquest was held in Newcastle on a man who fell backwards on to his head after being butted in a fight. About fourteen hours after admission to hospital he stopped breathing and was connected to an artificial respirator. Twenty-four hours later, with his wife's consent, a kidney was removed and grafted into another man. After the nephrectomy the respirator was disconnected and it was found that

---

[24] H. Hamlin, "Life or Death by EEG," *British Medical Journal* (1963), 2:394. This case was also reported in the *Journal of the American Medical Association* (1964), 190:112-14 and discussed by Halley and Harvey, "Medical and Legal Definitions of Death," pp. 103-4.

[25] E.D.R.S. and G.L.B.T., "The Moment of Death: Re Potter," *Medico-Legal Journal* (1963), 31:195. Cited by Louisell, in *Ethics in Medical Progress*, pp. 92-93.

there was no spontaneous respiration or circulation of the blood. A medical witness said that the man had virtually died at the time when he was put on the respirator, although it would be legally correct to say that death did not occur until 24 hours later, when breathing and the heart beat had ceased.

The cause of death was cerebral damage associated with a fractured skull. A neurosurgeon said that there was no hope of survival from the brain injury and that the patient was only put on the respirator because a kidney was wanted for transplanting. The recipient of the kidney died three weeks later. The assailant was commited for trial by the Coroner after a jury's verdict of manslaughter. The Coronor had consented to the removal of the kidney in accordance with the Human Tissue Act, 1961, section 1 (5) and the jury found that this had not contributed to death.[26]

In subsequent proceedings in the Magistrates Court, Potter's assailant was convicted on a reduced charge of common assault.

It is difficult, in view of the reports of this case, to say with any certainty *when* Mr. Potter died; that is, it is difficult to be precise unless one of several possible criteria is isolated as definitive of death. According to the attending physician, there were at least two kinds of death and different times assigned to each: medical death on June 16 and legal death on June 17. The neurologist and pathologist seemed satisfied that death occurred on June 16. But the coroner, in what must be the most astounding of all the opinions, held that the patient was alive at the time of the operation but that the operation did not contribute to his death, nor had the doctors committed any offense.

What this case indicates most clearly is that at present we simply do not have a uniform operational definition of death; one may be evolving, but the gap between heart death and brain death has not yet been bridged in any generally acceptable way.

[26] The relevant paragraphs from the Human Tissue Act, 1961, are in section 1: "(4) No such removal shall be effected except by a fully registered medical practitioner, who must have satisfied himself by personal examination of the body that life is extinct. (5) Where a person has reason to believe that an inquest may be required to be held on any body or that a post-mortem examination of any body may be required by the coroner, he shall not, except with the consent of the coroner,—(a) give an authority under this section in respect of the body; or (b) act on such an authority given by any other person."

That this will continue to provoke impassioned debate is manifest in view of almost worldwide persistence in heart transplantation; for the fact is that most cardiac homografting is conducted under circumstances quite similar to those in the Potter case. Indeed, the organ recipient in the Potter case could have needed a heart instead of a kidney and had that operation performed on grounds identical to the one that was performed. In that event, however, and supposing heart death to be definitive, the coroner's jury would have had to consider a verdict of murder rather than man-slaughter; and that question would have been compounded by the fact that the alleged victim's heart was still beating, but in the body of another person!

Five years after the Potter case, precisely this bizarre situation *almost* confronted authorities in Houston, Texas. On April 23, 1968, thirty-six-year-old Clarence A. Nicks received head injuries, from a beating in a Houston bar, severe enough to register a flat EEG. On May 7, St. Luke's Hospital announced that Nicks had died and that his heart had been transplanted into the body of sixty-two-year-old John M. Stuckwish. Harris County Medical Examiner, Dr. Joseph A. Jachmiczyk, reportedly cautioned against removing Nicks' heart "because he was the victim of a homicide." Jachmiczyk added that his caution was not "related to any ques-tion of whether Mr. Nicks was dead at the time of the transplant" but that "removal of the heart might affect the evidence in any court action that might result from the death of Mr. Nicks." [27] Despite the medical examiner's reassurance that Nicks was certain-ly dead at the time of transplant, the reference to evidence doubt-less had bearing upon whether, under Texas law, the "decedent" fully met the specific criteria for being pronounced dead: for Nicks' heart still beat, albeit in the body of another person! Texas jurists—I think unfortunately for both them and us—were spared the obvious dilemma by Stuckwish's death a week following the transplant; and Nicks' assailants were duly indicted on a charge of homicide. I have no doubt, however, that this specter will return to haunt us. The likelihood is that we will not face this matter until we are forced to; and when that happens, passion will vie

[27] *New York Times*, May 8, 1968.

with reason, and emotion with intellect, for resolution of an issue that demands our most sober and sane reflection.

The effective consequence of not having a uniform operational definition of death is what theologians would call *anomie*, literally "without law." This does not mean that there are no statutes which define death; but it does mean, as we have seen, that innovations in biomedical support systems have liberated the old criteria and that existing statutory definitions are more or less mooted, with the practical result that different doctors employ different criteria for defining and pronouncing death. To be sure, this situation presents the heightened possibility of legal prosecution to doctors themselves, but that would appear to be a remote probability in view of historical precedent. More serious is the inequality in patient care that appears to be the unavoidable precondition of evolving a new consensus. There are doubtless hundreds, and perhaps thousands, of patients in neurological and other hospital services who are now being mechanically metabolized by artificial means and who have no serious medical expectation of recovery. In order to spare these patients needless extension of their distress, their families needless anxiety and expense, hospital personnel and facilities needless consumption of skill and resource, and waiting patients needless delay in receiving attention—for all these and other worthy reasons we desperately need to know and agree when further possibility of life recovery has been exhausted and artificial means of death deferment may be terminated.

V

The principle is already well established, in both law and theological ethics as well as medicine, that physicians are obligated to use all "ordinary" means to preserve and prolong life but that their decision to apply "extraordinary" means in a given case is optional and discretionary. Statutes are sufficiently vague on the distinction between ordinary and extraordinary, so that judicial decision normally depends on what doctors customarily do. Roman Catholic theologians are more specific: ordinary means are "all medicines, treatments and operations which offer a reasonable hope of benefit, and which can be obtained and used without excessive expense, pain or other inconvenience"; extraordinary means, on the other hand, are those resources and appliances which would involve "excessive expense, pain, or other inconvenience" and not offer "reasonable hope of benefit." [28] Doctors tend to be a bit more pragmatic: ordinary means are established medical and surgical procedures appropriate to a given illness within the limits of availability; extraordinary means are those procedures (including medicines) which are incompletely established, frankly experimental, or bizarre.[29] Among all the disciplines it is recognized that the distinction is relative and that it will vary with time, place, and situation. In the end, physicians themselves must be the primary arbiters of the distinction, although the principle itself is grounded in common sense.

Much more difficult to sort out is a further distinction which applies to decisions affecting the termination of life (or the acceleration of death), and this is the subtle and delicate discrimination between direct and indirect methods. Several factors impinge upon the moral and professional logic of this distinction. Among them is a principle which derives from both the Hippocratic Oath ("I will follow that method of treatment which, according to my ability and judgment, I consider for the benefit of my patients, and abstain from whatever is deleterious and mischievous. I will give no deadly medicine to anyone if asked, nor suggest any such counsel") and the Judeo-Christian tradition ("Thou shalt not kill") that a doctor may not actively and deliberately kill his patient. On the other hand, both law and theology acknowledge that a doctor may legitimately abstain from acting to prevent death or even contribute indirectly to death.

Illustrative of the murky and fragile state of the law in these matters is the way in which George Fletcher applies the distinction in his article, "Legal Aspects of the Decision Not to Prolong Life." The fundamental question, according to Fletcher, is two-

[28] Gerald Kelly, "The Duty to Preserve Life," *Theological Studies* (1951), 12:550.

[29] J. C. Ford and J. E. Drew, "Advising Radical Surgery: A Problem in Medical Morality," *Journal of the American Medical Association* (1953), 151:711-16.

fold: (1) what is the relationship between the doctor and the sick or injured person, and (2) does the doctor's conduct fall in the category of "act" or "omission"? These queries interrelate in determination of the doctor's legal duty and liability. If the doctor's conduct is determined to be an "omission," the relationship between himself and the sick or injured person is all-controlling; if, on the other hand, the doctor's conduct is determined to be an "act," the relationship is irrelevant. What this seems to mean practically is that a doctor is criminally and civilly liable for a patient who justifiably relies on him for medical attention, but not similarly liable for a "stranger." Moreover, this way of stating the matter appears to mean that an "act" by a doctor constitutes *ipso facto* a doctor-patient relationship, even though the one acted toward or upon is a "stranger," which, in turn, makes the doctor liable. Thus, refusing to answer a patient's call is an "act" (legally interpreted) while refusing to respond to a stranger's call is an "omission." [30]

Furthermore, Fletcher contends that the distinction between "act" and "omission" is roughly analogous to the difference between "causing" and "permitting." Moreover, he argues that withdrawing instrumental support (as, for example, by turning off a respirator) from a dying patient simply permits death to occur and is thus denominated an "omission."

To this point I do not profess to understand, but only report, this argument. One impression does, however, begin to emerge from Fletcher's turgid linguistic analysis, and a clue to it is provided in the following sentences: "The use of the term 'prolongation of life' builds on the same perception of reality that prompts us to say that turning off the respirator is an activity permitting death to occur, rather than causing death. And that basic perception is that using the respirator interferes artificially in the pattern of [natural] events." [31] One suspects, in view of this kind of

[30] The exception to this general rule occurs in those states where "Good Samaritan" statutes have been enacted. These laws permit, but do not require, doctors to attend to "strangers" (for example, accident victims) without incurring customary liability for them as patients.

[31] George P. Fletcher, "Legal Aspects of the Decision Not to Prolong Life," p. 67.

language, that what Fletcher really signifies by "act" is personal and professional interference with natural processes and that "omission," correspondingly, means the abdication of further personal and professional responsibility to a vague kind of naturalistic determinism. That this approach has long been the *modus operandi* of Western law and medicine (and often theology as well) is not at issue; whether it should continue to be so is a primary question we have pursued throughout these chapters.

We can bracket the larger philosophical and theological problem just now and return to a practical application of Fletcher's analysis. What of those situations in which the doctor is confronted with the decision whether to act or not to act? The decision to prolong or not to prolong life—or to defer or accelerate death—is just such a situation. Fletcher argues that in the case of a patient who has clearly expressed to his physician the wish that everything possible be done to keep him alive, even when there is no medical hope of recovery, the doctor is legally obligated to employ every medical means at his disposal to do just that. To act contrary to this expressed wish or to omit to act toward its implementation would make the doctor legally liable. In another case, however, in which there is no explicit instruction from the patient, it is reasonable to suppose that the patient's expectations for his care are based on the customary practices of the time. "Thus," says Fletcher, "we have come full circle. We began the inquiry by asking: is it legally permissible for doctors to turn off respirators used to prolong the life of doomed patients? And the answer after our tortuous journey is simply this: it all depends on what doctors customarily do. The law is sometimes no more precise than that." [32]

David Daube, Regius Professor of Civil Law at Oxford University, has taken a considerably more rigorous view of the limits imposed by law upon this aspect of medical practice. Arguing that questions of when it is in order to discontinue life-prolonging measures should not be confused with the question of when a man is dead, Daube says: "Under the classical definition of death, which should not be lightly discarded, an irreversibly unconscious

[32] *Ibid.*, p. 68.

person whose life depends on a machine is still alive. The doctor may be right to stop the machine and let him die. But until death occurs, interference with his body is illicit: it is not a corpse." [33] Daube's assessment of this situation embraces two suppositions, neither of which can any longer claim to be incontrovertible but both of which are widely held: (1) that cessation of spontaneous cardiopulmonary activity is prerequisite to death, and (2) that a direct action which has as its primary intention the termination of human life is murder.

We have already indicated that considerable dubiety surrounds the first of these suppositions; now a brief comment is in order with respect to the second. In the statutes defining first-degree murder in the United States, two conditions are required: premeditation and malice. The absurdity of this legal fiction (which presumes that if human life be taken intentionally and with forethought, it must correspondingly be taken with hatred and enmity) is demonstrated, however, both by criminological and sociopsychological studies which show that the majority of malicious killings are not premeditated, and by the peculiar circumstances which circumscribe the management of dying patients. I do not think that it either can or should be held, as though it were irreversible logic, that every deliberate termination of life is accompanied by malevolence as an inexorable correlate of premeditation. No one can doubt, of course, that there are instances of killing in which premeditation and malice are frankly joined; but what I dissent from is the view that malice is a function of premeditation and that if one kills intentionally he also, by defintion, kills hatefully.

Anyone familiar with the most rudimentary psychological insights will appreciate that a decision to terminate the life (and, incidentally, the pain) of an incurably diseased and distressed patient is equivocal and ambiguous. Similarly, anyone familiar with the most elementary ethical perceptions knows that no decision, and surely one of great significance, is without doubt and risk. Families might be selfishly motivated; so may be doctors

[33] David Daube, in *Ethics in Medical Progress*, p. 191.

and nurses; even the patient himself may be pathologically depressed or crazed by pain. But a straightforward admission of these ingredients in the decision-making process does not prove "beyond a reasonable doubt" that an intentional choice for death is a hateful and unloving act. Meantime, however, the laws remain unchanged; and their simplistic formulation contributes to injustice, hypocrisy, and the invention of ever more sophisticated artifice and circumvention.

Mrs. Katie Roberts was a helpless invalid who suffered from multiple sclerosis. During the summer of 1918 she attempted suicide by taking carbolic acid. She was examined in February, 1919, by her doctor, who observed that she was bedridden and practically helpless, that her body was wasted and showed signs of a protracted illness, and that she had the rapid pulse, hesitating and singsong speech, and other outward manifestations of multiple sclerosis. The doctor concluded that Mrs. Roberts' case was incurable but nevertheless sent her to a hospital. After thirty days in the hospital Mrs. Roberts was discharged. Two months later she urged her husband to mix a quantity of Paris green (aceto-arsenite) and water for her. Mr. Roberts mixed the poison and placed it on a chair near his wife's bed; Mrs. Roberts drank the poison and died within a few hours. Mr. Roberts was convicted of murder in the first degree and sentenced to life imprisonment.[34]

More recently, Mrs. Alice Waskin was admitted to the emergency room of Chicago's Wesley Memorial Hospital on August 7, 1968, in a deep coma and near death from an overdose of sleeping pills. She was a victim of leukemia and in recent weeks had complained bitterly of her pain. On August 8, while Mrs. Waskin lay in the hospital's intensive care unit, her twenty-four-year-old son, Robert, kissed her and then fired two bullets into her head. During Robert Waskin's trial on a charge of first-degree murder, one group of expert witnesses testified that he appeared calm and normal on the day of the slaying; another group of expert witnesses testified that anyone acting under such stresses would be

[34] *People* v. *Roberts*, 211 *Michigan Reports* 187, 178 *Northwestern Reporter* 690 (1920).

suffering a severe mental depression, and that Waskin probably did not know that what he was doing was wrong. On January 24, 1969, a jury of eight men and four women required only forty minutes and one ballot to find Robert Waskin not guilty by reason of temporary insanity.[35]

These cases, which could be multiplied many times, are not cited in order to raise the question of the legal guilt or innocence of particular individuals; that is a matter, in a society governed by laws, for the courts. What is clear from these cases and our entire discussion, however, is that there are urgent prior questions about our understandings of life and death, and the adequacy of current statutory formulations to express them, that cry out for serious and sustained attention. To accept intellectually that there *is* an appropriate time to die carries with it a concomitant responsibility to try to say, however tentatively and provisionally in view of the modern situation, *when* that time is; otherwise our judgments of those who venture to act on this postulate are liable to be arbitrary, and our cerebral commitments will tend to eventuate in practical self-delusion and hypocrisy. Sooner or later we must come to grips with at least some of the hard questions and practical implications that confront us; or frankly admit that we really believe human mastery over life and death to be demonic, that nature's way is God's way, and abandon further attempts at controlling human destiny. One hopeful sign is indicated by the National Conference of Commissioners on Uniform State Laws, which is currently engaged in studying certain statutes and drafting uniform codes. Given the proliferation of state laws, together with the powers reserved to states by the Constitution, the Commissioners have undertaken an awesome task. Still, it is not too much to hope that this group or some other like it will soon address the broad range of statutes affecting the definition and criteria of death which are in immediate need of reexamination in light of current developments in science and technology.

[35] See Jerry Lipson, "Mrs. Waskin Overdose Told," *Chicago Daily News*, January 25, 1969; and "Freed Mercy Killer Toasts 'Life,' " *Chicago Daily News*, January 27, 1969. See also Luis Kutner, "Due Process of Euthanasia," *Indiana Law Journal* (1969) 44:539 ff.

VI

It is no more within the special competence of theologians than of lawyers to say *when* death has occurred; that is a judgment, as we all probably agree, that is appropriate to physicians. But the judgment that death has occurred is informed by a number of considerations, of which medical diagnosis is only one and to which theology and law can contribute their own distinctive resources. We have already indicated that statutory regulations are among the factors which describe the conditions prerequisite to pronouncing death; now we must add that there are religious considerations for the meaning, purpose, and value of human life which also influence the judgment that death has occurred. Were this chapter a general examination of the entire matrix of factors which impinge on the decision, we would also consider public opinion, experimental priorities, and other ancillary areas; but we are chiefly concerned with the disciplines of medicine, law, and theology, and it is especially within this interdisciplinary context that increasing numbers of theologians and lawyers are unwilling to accept the claim of some (not all!) doctors that the definition and criteria of death are exclusively within the province, and are therefore the prerogative, of the medical profession.

It deserves emphasis that it is at the point of conceptual clarity, and not technical execution of judgment, that such interprofessional and interdisciplinary collaboration and feedback are both most urgent and appropriate. Particularly in view of the broad range of competing and sometimes conflicting opinions which have emerged from medical research and biomedical technology, both theologians and lawyers share with doctors a suitable interest in trying to sort out a consensus with respect to where the priorities lie. That a number of different signs, heretofore unknown or too imprecise to employ, are now in the picture, and that the prominence attributed to any one of them tends inevitably to affect the care and treatment of human beings, suffices to engender fitting theological interest in these questions. Beyond this, however, Christian moralists are concerned with relationships between character and conduct, belief and behavior, and therefore have immense professional interest in the dilemma

151

which occurs when, in decisions affecting the life and death of patients, a doctor discovers his own conscience to be on a collision course with his profession's clearly enunciated creed and the law's certain mandate.

Two concerns generally characterize authentic Christian moral reflection: (1) to perceive as clearly as possible God's will, as this is manifest in Jesus Christ, and to relate that will to the conduct of human affairs; and (2) to assess the coherence and congeniality between particular actions and affirmed values. Because what we *do* effectively communicates our *operative beliefs*, because *is*-ness is a function of our perception of *ought*-ness, moralists ask what values are signified by behavior and whether, with reference to both God and the situation, they are appropriate. It sometimes happens that the relatively "right" action is done, but for the wrong reason; just as sometimes the relatively "wrong" action is premised on the right values. The moralists' task is to assist in discriminating among these relative alternatives.

The immediate values at issue in consideration of life-prolongation or death-acceleration have to do with the worth we attach to human life, so let us be clear about the value of life at the outset. It is a mistake to suppose that the basis for a Christian view of human life lies in an attribution of absolute value to life as such. Christians have typically held that human life is a gift from God, and therefore ultimately subject to him. Moreover, the entire spectrum of human events—from birth to death, with all its satisfactions and disappointments and successes and failures—has traditionally been ascribed to God's will. This or that happened as an effective consequence of God's causative will—a couple is fecund or infertile, a child is mentally retarded or precocious, a nation wins or loses a war, a man dies peacefully in his sleep or lives out his last days in protracted pain and distress—and all these apparent contradictions have been plausible to Christians at one or another time because belief in the sovereignty of God was interpreted as a cause-and-effect correlation between God's will and human events.

We have already shown that this kind of reasoning produced a body of doctrine which tends to identify the will of God with what is "natural," and that the professions of medicine and law together with theology adopted such a rationale as the basis of moral codes. Thus, law in the Western tradition is very much concerned with what it takes to be "natural rights," formulating statutes for their protection; and medicine has thought of itself as a servant of natural processes, correcting and curing what it takes to be unnatural anomalies in the human body (which is itself a "natural" organism). To be sure, this has not been, especially since the Renaissance, a purely reflective action; and doctors and lawyers, as well as theologians, have become increasingly aware that their perceptions of what is "natural" are influenced by many factors which permit, indeed oblige, them somehow to transcend the naked boundaries of natural cause and effect. So the law acknowledges that social and political organization qualifies so-called natural rights; and doctors surely know that every therapeutic measure, from giving aspirin to performing delicate brain surgery, interferes with bare natural processes. In short, both law and medicine have a metaphysic, i.e., an *idea* of what nature intends that is not always deduced from a simple observation of the way things happen "naturally" to be.

That this is so comes as no surprise to any man who has reflected on the relationship between what he does and why he does it. In the daily round of every sensitive person the question recurs again and again: What must or should I do? That is the *moral* question; and the sum of the answers given to that question constitutes a set of morals. But the question "What must I do?" raises a logically prior question, and that is, "Where do I look to find out what I should do? That is the *ethical* question; and the sum of the answers given to that question constitutes one's ethics or value postulates. Whereas morals are immediately concerned with action, ethics is the discipline of self-conscious reflection upon various moral alternatives. Every moral judgment is therefore rooted in a certain value; and the value itself is finally undemonstrable, an *a priori* judgment that in religious language might be called a "faith assumption." For Christians the ultimate reality, the *a priori* if you like, is the God whom Jesus revealed; and it is this God who is the ground of human life and the proper referent of all human action and thought. Of course, non-Christians affirm other ultimate referents. The point, withal, is that all men, either implicitly or explicitly, ask these questions and answer them in a way that is more or less personally satisfactory. The role of the Christian theologian, then, in considerations of human life and human death, is to articulate as clearly and convincingly as possible how, with reference to the values which derive from Christian faith, we can deal with these events and actions.

Theology, no less than law and medicine, has surely contributed to the notion that all human species life is immune from direct aggression and that each life is equal in value to every other life. Moreover, theologians have conventionally distinguished between direct and indirect actions in ways that congenially parallel the lawyer's distinction between act and omission or "causing" and "permitting," and the doctor's distinction between "prolonging life" and "allowing to die." All three disciplines are heavily indebted historically to natural law, and it is therefore not surprising that all have tended to arrive at fundamentally the same conclusions.

We saw earlier, in the discussion of abortion, that traditional Christian teaching prohibits *direct* aggression against nascent life on the grounds that all life is a gift from God, endowed by him with a soul, and wholly at his disposal. Every human-species being is therefore supposed to enjoy an inherent and inalienable right to life, and from some imprecise moment onward—fertilization, blastocyst, nidation, or whatever—this is said to be inviolable. We also noted in that context, however, that there are some instances in which *indirect* abortion is both permitted and justified by theologians under the rule of double-effect. There are serious difficulties and deficiencies in this view, and particularly with the rule of double-effect; but similar reasoning characterizes the thought of many theologians (predominantly, but not exclusively, Roman Catholic) with respect to the care and management of terminally ill or irremediably injured patients.

Roman Catholic moralists who comment on these matters, usually under the heading of "euthanasia," are unanimous in their absolute condemnation of any action which has as its primary intention the direct killing (as distinguished from hastening the dying process) of an incurably ill or injured patient, even when this action may have been requested by the patient himself. Ac-

154

companing this general prohibition, however, is qualified approval—i.e., qualified by the rule of double-effect—of indirect actions which may shorten life and accelerate death. Thus, Bernard Häring acknowledges that "the end may possibly be hastened slightly accidentally and indirectly." [36] And Henry Davis, a Jesuit professor of moral theology, concurs: "If acute pain must be relieved, and if the patient is already prepared by all spiritual means to die, it appears to be morally right to employ drugs to relieve pain and incidentally to take away consciousness." [37]

Papal sanction for the view that a patient's life may be indirectly abbreviated was given by Pius XII in an address on February 24, 1957:

If there exists no direct or causal link, either through the will of interested parties or by the nature of things, between the induced unconsciousness and the shortening of life—as would be the case if the suppression of the pain could be obtained only by the shortening of life; and if, on the other hand, the actual administration of drugs brings about two distinct effects, the one the relief of pain, the other the shortening of life, the action is lawful. It is necessary, however, to observe whether there is between these two effects, a reasonable proportion, and if the advantages of the one compensate for the disadvantages of the other.[38]

That direct killing is an illicit interference with human life is certainly one of the assumptions which informs this position; but human life does not constitute an absolute value for Roman Catholics, as sanctions for just war and capital punishment eloquently attest and as the rule of double-effect makes abundantly clear. What is actually more basic to this argument is the category of *innocence* which serves to qualify the sanctity of human life. The prohibition in Catholic teaching applies to direct killing of innocent life. Just war is defended when one nation is threatened by the aggression of another nation, and capital punishment is approved for those whose natural rights are forfeited by the

[36] *The Law of Christ*, III, 213.
[37] Henry Davis, *Moral and Pastoral Theology*, II, 196. Earlier in the same paragraph Davis defines euthanasia as "an euphemism for the deliberate taking away of the consciousness of another, so that it will not return before death."
[38] *Acta Apostolicae Sedis*, 49:146.

commission and conviction of a capital crime. Innocence is thus interpreted to mean personal guiltlessness with respect to aggression against the common good or another individual; and, in the practical circumstance of moral alternatives, the category thereby becomes a juridical concept. Where natural innocence is displaced by juridical guilt, there is no ethical objection to employing direct action for the termination of life.

I doubt, however, that innocence, as a value referent, can be so unambiguously translated into such specific behavioral modes. Who, after all, is innocent and from whence does innocence derive? To apply a juridical concept of innocence finally begs the moral question, an example of which is the case of the condemned criminal who falls ill and for whom every medical assistance is provided (at cost to the state!) in order that he recover and be healthy at the time of his execution. Of course this is an exceptional and only occasional situation; but it is not so far removed *morally* from the obverse situation in which competent medical diagnosis is of terminal illness or irremediable injury and no action is permitted, even when requested by the patient, which will directly accelerate death.

Beyond this aspect of the problem, it deserves asking whether we can say without equivocation that doctors who refuse to allow an accident victim to die (for example, one whose brain is destroyed) are not agressors against the well-being of the patient's family and *all* their resources so long as the patient's death is artificially postponed? Or that the hundreds of hours and millions of dollars expended in the care of mechanically metabolized human organisms, for whom there is no real medical hope of recovery, do not constitute in some sense an assault upon the common good? I do not mean to imply, by raising these questions, that we should have no hesitancy about assisting these people to die or killing them directly; I only wish to argue that the moral calculus is not finally determinable by any single factor—not even innocence—and that it is therefore important that all the variables in the mix be self-consciously sorted out, assessed, and assigned a place of relative priority according to their respective bearing on the decision-making moment.

In addition, there is surely a direct and causal link between induced unconsciousness and the shortening of life when pain can be relieved only by the administration of drugs which knowingly abbreviate life. When this is so, it is self-deluding to ignore the obvious relationship between narcosis and death-acceleration or to obscure it by sophisticated word games. Glanville Williams has articulated the subtle moral deception to which the rule of double effect is prey:

> It is altogether too artificial to say that a doctor who gives an overdose of a narcotic having in the forefront of his mind the aim of ending his patient's existence is guilty of sin, while a doctor who gives the same overdose in the same circumstances in order to relieve pain is not guilty of sin, provided that he keeps his mind steadily off the consequences which his professional training teaches him is inevitable, namely the death of his patient. When you know that your conduct will have two consequences, one in itself good and one in itself evil, you are compelled as a moral agent to choose between acting and not acting by making a judgment of value, that is to say by deciding whether the good is more to be desired than the evil is to be avoided. If this is what the principle of double effect means, well and good; but if it means that the necessity of making a choice of values can be avoided merely by keeping your mind off one of the consequences, it can only encourage a hypocritical attitude towards moral problems.[39]

Roman Catholic theologians are not alone in arguing that there is a sharp moral distinction to be made between direct actions which intend and cause death and indirect actions which allow, and in some cases hasten, death. Dietrich Bonhoeffer and Karl Barth are representative of those Protestant theologians who hold that it is for God alone to make an end of human life and that any direct action taken against the lives of the sick or incurably infirm is tantamount to murder.

"The question of principle is this," says Bonhoeffer, "is it permissible to destroy painlessly an innocent life which is no longer worth living?" Without explicating what he means by phrases like "innocent life" and "no longer worth living," Bonhoeffer states firmly "as a matter of principle" that a decision to kill directly can never be taken as one among several possibilities: it is either an "unconditional necessity," in which case the killing

[39] Glanville Williams, *The Sanctity of Life*, pp. 321-22.

must be done irrespective of all the arguments against it, or an "arbitrary killing," in which case it is murder. Bonhoeffer then reduces to two the several arguments usually put forward in defense of direct euthanasia: (1) consideration for the incurably sick and painwracked patient, and (2) consideration for the healthy. The first of these is rejected because Bonhoeffer doubts that patients in intense pain can make a valid voluntary request for their own death; the second is repudiated because of its alleged utilitarian, rather than theocentric, value for life. Underlying both arguments, but again unexplained, is an assumption that there is a morally significant difference between killing and allowing to die.[40]

Bonhoeffer's *Ethics*, as those familiar with his life and untimely death know, is fragmentary and incomplete; had he lived to complete his work, some sections might have been expanded and some of the ambiguous phrases and assumptions clarified. On the other hand, it is well known that Bonhoeffer's writing did not proceed sequentially or systematically and that the *Ethics*, in particular, was composed of a number of separate studies. Pervasive themes are consequently detectable in a way that specific meanings are not, and it is from these themes that we get a clue as to the overarching rationale which informed his writing. Two of these are definitely reflected in Bonhoeffer's brief comments on human life and death: (1) that God alone is the author and finisher of life, and (2) that in the sight of God there is no life that is not worth living.[41]

It is not gratuitous to observe that had Bonhoeffer applied these principles rigorously to his own life, he might not have been executed by the Nazis for the part he played in an assassination plot against Hitler. That he could take this action and hold these views of the sanctity of life, however, is symptomatic of the dualism in his ethics. And that, in the final analysis, he denominates "innocence" as the determinative category for the prohibition against deliberate destruction of life[42] renders his appeal to a

[40] Bonhoeffer, *Ethics*, pp. 116-20.
[41] See esp. *Ibid.*, p. 119.
[42] Cf. *Ibid.*, pp. 121-22.

single criterion as morally problematic as Roman Catholic casuistry. The systematic extermination of certain classes of persons in Germany in the 1930's and early 1940's was doubtless known to Bonhoeffer and may largely account for the absolutely uncompromising position which he took toward euthanasia.[43] Under similar circumstances, odds are that a morally sensitive person would adopt the same attitude. But the circumstance of "the man who is incurably sick and for the grievousness of his suffering demands the deliberate termination of his life by some humane form of death" is not the same as compulsory and involuntary euthanasia, and that is the nub of *our* problem: can a man legitimately exercise any control over the manner and time of his death? Bonhoeffer's answer is that "the question regarding euthanasia must be answered in the negative." [44]

When we examined Karl Barth's views on direct abortion, it developed that his exception to an otherwise general prohibition of abortion was related to those situations in which two lives, the mother's and the fetus', were in conflict: "For all concerned, what must be at stake must be life against life, *nothing other nor less*, if the decision is not to be a wrong decision and the resultant action murder either of the child or the mother." [45] At the other pole of the human life cycle, however, there does not appear to be

[43] The "Law for the Prevention of Hereditarily Diseased Posterity" was promulgated in July, 1933; and in March, 1934, a comprehensive commentary on this law was issued. These, in turn, led to compulsory euthanasia of the incurably insane and systematic extermination of certain races (Poles, Russians, Jews, gypsies) who were declared to be inferior. For a comprehensive summary of euthanasia procedures, together with accounts of various German court proceedings, see Alice Platen-Hallermund, *Die Tötung Geisteskranker in Deutschland* (Frankfurt am Main: Frankfurter Hefte Verlag, 1948). Hitler's euthanasia decree, signed September 1, 1939, authorized that certain physicians be designated in order "that persons who, according to human judgment, are incurable can, upon a most careful diagnosis of their condition of sickness, be accorded a mercy death." (Cited in A. Mitscherlich and F. Mielke, *The Death Doctors*, trans. James Cleugh [London: Elek Books, 1962], pp. 235-36.) The gassing of mentally afflicted adults was terminated in the autumn of 1941, by which time an estimated 100,000 persons had been killed; but deformed and idiotic children continued to be liquidated until the end of the war.

[44] *Ethics*, pp. 117, 121.

[45] *Church Dogmatics*, III/4, 422. Italics added.

ETHICS AND THE NEW MEDICINE

another life in *direct* and *immediate* competition, and Barth here maintains that there is no alternative but to respect life by preserving it. Commenting on the question whether society has the right to declare certain sick people unfit to live—which, in our terms of reference, is compulsory euthanasia—Barth answers with "an unequivocal No. This is a type of killing which can be regarded only as murder, i.e., as a wicked usurpation of God's sovereign right over life and death." [46]

As for voluntary euthanasia—when, at a certain stage of treatment, medical resources are exhausted and both the patient and his family request an end to suffering and help to die—Barth grants that "tempting questions" are raised; but "for all their impressiveness, they contain too much sophistry for those who are directed by the command of God to be able to give an affirmative answer." The sum of the matter, as regards both voluntary and compulsory termination of human life by direct means, is succinctly stated in the same paragraph: "The central insight in this whole complex of problems is that it is for God and God alone to make an end of human life, and that man should help in this only when he has a specific and clear command from God." [47]

The final clause in that sentence might suggest that Barth does indeed leave open the possibility of a "specific clear command from God" in the exceptional case. In the interlinear note which concludes the section on euthanasia he introduces that possibility, immediately rejects it, and then ends the discussion with five trenchant sentences which leave the reader dangling on the dialectical tightrope:

Yet in this connexion, the question also arises whether this kind of artificial prolongation of life does not amount to human arrogance in the opposite direction, whether the fulfillment of medical duty does not threaten to become fanaticism, reason folly, and the required assisting of human life a forbidden torturing of it. A case is at least conceivable in which a doctor might have to recoil from this prolongation of life no less than from its arbitrary shortening. We must await further developments in this sphere to get a clear general picture. But

[46] *Ibid.*, p. 423.
[47] *Ibid.*, p. 425.

160

it may well be that in this special sphere we do have a kind of exceptional case. For it is not now a question of arbitrary euthanasia; it is a question of the respect which may be claimed by even the dying life as such.[48]

Advocates of direct euthanasia, however voluntary, will nevertheless look in vain for support from Barth. Certainly the greater weight of the evidence of his total discussion does not lend encouragement to the notion that there is, in fact, any situation which can qualify as the exceptional case. In addition, since Barth did not define "life against life" in such a way as to embrace indirect and proximate, as well as direct and immediate, conflict, there is no reasonable way to infer support from his argument when plainly, on his terms, only one life is at issue in cases affecting the terminally ill or irremediably injured patient. One suspects, on reflection, that the provocative issues raised in Barth's final note deserve considerably more urgent and thorough attention than he himself supposed.

Paul Ramsey also defends the general prohibition against direct action which causes or assists human dying and argues that we cannot exceed the moral boundaries of allowing to die: "Every effort should be made to save a patient, no matter how bad off he seems to a static diagnosis. But only up to a point, however difficult it may be to draw this line and to say when this particular patient's dying has taken irreversible control. . . . This means that medical conscience must learn to be willing to begin treatment and then to stop it." [49] Ramsey does not venture to say, however, *when* this decision may be taken or *where* the point is that this line should be drawn. That is the doctor's judgment. Ramsey also appreciates that these are choices which depend heavily upon the distinction between ordinary and extraordinary means and, more important, that this is a very relative distinction which is contingent upon too many factors to allow precise and stationary definition. Withal, he is not reluctant to call into question the morality of relentless and unqualified efforts to prolong life; neither is he convinced that everything that can be done ought

[48] *Ibid.*, p. 427.
[49] Ramsey, "Some Terms of Reference for the Abortion Debate."

to be done in every case to preserve life. In the end, however, we are left again with Barth's vexing question and rather indefinite instruction as to how we can discriminate between saving life and torturing it, how medical duty can be responsible without being arrogant, how one goes about deciding whether "to intervene upon the scientific interventions that save life, to negate some of the negative consequences of the practice of saving life." [50]

That all Protestant theologians do not share the general position represented by Bonhoeffer and Barth should not be very surprising. Among the proponents of the moral legitimacy of voluntary euthanasia (no Christian theologian to my knowledge endorses or advocates compulsory euthanasia), none is perhaps better known than Joseph Fletcher, whose book *Morals and Medicine* has become something of a landmark in Protestant theological reflection on medical ethics. Unlike Bonhoeffer and Barth, Fletcher's starting point is not with a doctrine of divine sovereignty or any notion that it is for God alone to make an end of human life. "Our principle of personal integrity," he says, "asserts that there is a place for the doctrine of human agency in the scheme of creation. . . . In any ethical outlook of religious faith, men are people and not puppets. It is a false humility or a subtle determinism which asks us to 'leave things in God's hands.' The worst forms of determinism and fatalism are spiritualistic, not materialistic. They are more often grounded in theistic religion than in humanism." [51]

Fletcher's ethics rest upon what he calls "a principle of freedom within responsibility" which entails

two negative *oughts*: (1) we ought not to submit willy-nilly to what is, to physical and physiological facts simply as they are, since to do so would be to be unfree; and (2) we ought not to ignore or disregard or flout what is, simply because it is unchosen, since to do so would be to be guilty of an unrealistic denial of human finitude and creaturehood and therefore irresponsible—toward both our natural necessities and our social obligations. [52]

[50] *Ibid.*
[51] *Morals and Medicine* p. 215.
[52] *Ibid.*, p. 213.

From this perspective Fletcher undertakes a moral analysis of the ways in which what he calls "customary morality" destroys human freedom and distorts human knowledge and thereby deprives man of the capacity to be a moral being.

The medical problem with euthanasia, as Fletcher rightly says, arises out of a logical contradiction in the Hippocratic Oath: doctors promise to relieve suffering and to prolong life, but these supposedly complementary duties often come into conflict. The moral problem arises when customary morality "condemns us to live, or to put it another way, destroys our moral being for the sake of just *being*." [53] The objections to voluntary euthanasia by customary morality—which range from arguments that this action is suicide, murder, and a violation of God's right to decide the moment of death to protests that the patient may miraculously recover and that physicians themselves do not want the procedure (i.e., intervening to stop their relentless interventions) to be legalized—are then examined by Fletcher; and one by one, both religious and medical items in the bill of particulars are methodically repudiated and set aside. Because the discussion is confined to voluntary euthanasia, or what Fletcher later calls "anti-dysthanasia" (literally, against bad death), he does not address the questions of eugenic euthanasia (for monstrosities or mental defectives at birth) or involuntary euthanasia (for those who are "burdens on the community").

His conclusion, in substance, is that the issue of voluntary euthanasia "is not one of life or death. The issue is which kind of death, an agonized or peaceful one. Shall we meet death in personal integrity or in personal disintegration? Should there be a moral or a demoralized end to mortal life?" To these rhetorical questions, Fletcher answers that "we are not as persons of moral stature to be ruled by ruthless and unreasoning physiology, but rather by reason and self-control." Implicit in this answer is his verdict that the supreme value is personality and that "the counter-Reformation version of the classical Natural Law, which in its new form so consistently subordinates human values to the law

[53] *Ibid.*, pp. 172, 176.

163

of nature, is a perversion of a moral norm into a physical or material norm." [54]

Fletcher's position moves toward liberating moral decision from the bondage of natural or supernatural cause-and-effect; and to that extent he offers the alternative of human decisional apparatus—freedom and knowledge—in matters affecting life and death. If the difficulties, however, with Catholic natural law and Protestant theocentrism are their tendencies to deprive man of responsibility for his choices and his future, the corresponding difficulty with Fletcher's humanistic personalism is that he credits too much to man's reason and self-control, and fails to take seriously enough those values for the conduct of human life which derive from theistic religion in general and Christian faith in particular. It is not necessary to discredit theism in favor of humanism in order to establish a viable relationship between the two; indeed, careful examination of every professed humanistic philosophy will reveal at least implicit theistic hypotheses and postulates underlying it. What is needed, therefore, is not only criticism of customary morality and the premises on which it is grounded, but a comprehensive and coherent ethics which articulates the relationship between what is perceived to be God's will and the manifold and sometimes chaotic contexts of human existence and action.

VII

This, in fact, is what the present and the preceding chapters have been about. Accordingly, the basic context I have espoused is both personal and interpersonal—understood theistically as a personal God who relates interpersonally. Moreover, I have claimed that the moral calculus which impinges upon all these issues, and now specifically the management of dying patients, is not determinable by a single, unambiguous value, but by clusters of value which, in a given case, constitute the fundamental variables from which choices and actions derive. Within this approach it has seemed both appropriate and arguable that human

[54] *Ibid., pp.* 208, 222.

life and human death must be comprehended personally and interpersonally as well as bodily-biologically. That is, bodily-biological life is understood to be preconditional to personal life, the necessary but not sufficient condition for the emergence and sustenance of personal life. The basic question which therefore concerns us is the question of personal life: if we have the necessary biological conditions, we can have personal life; if, on the other hand, we do not have the necessary biological conditions—foremost among which is a functioning brain in a human body—we may have biological activity without personal life. Finally, as I tried to show in the conclusion to Chapter I, the context I have advocated also includes an eschatological perspective of personal and interpersonal life with new forms, conditions, and possibilities of bodily life.

There is, I think, increasing evidence for the claim that we need to face *directly* and *promptly* the consequences of decisions for action or inaction, whether "direct" or "indirect," and to view these consequences through a personal as well as biological conception of human life and human death. Facing these issues in these ways, we cannot then avoid confronting the inadequacy of artificial, self-deceptive distinctions which effectively disguise the real issues at stake in these decisions. Theologians, especially, must insist that the management of terminal illness or injury sustain, *as far as possible*, the personal dignity and integrity of the patient, together with the interpersonal values of the relationships between the patient and larger contexts of other persons, particularly the immediate family. Functionally, this means that theologians, together with other professionals involved in these decisions, must insist upon an open and thorough consideration of *all* the options for the management of terminally ill or irremediably injured patients as *live* options.

Perhaps the most succinct and appropriate way to combine tentativeness of statement with finality of commitment, at least as this bears upon issues of this sort, is to say candidly and forthrightly that if there is sufficient indication of brain death, or brain damage to the extent of irreversibile loss of consciousness and function, we are no longer dealing in any way with a person. The person as a person is dead so far as any medical access is concerned; [55] moreover, the person is also dead so far as any personal access is concerned—i.e., in relation to us and us to him. Under these circumstances we are then dealing with an unburied corpse; and, following Daube's proposals,[56] we can therefore use the cadaver both in the service of the living and in ways that are medically, legally, and ethically acceptable—including, I would think, preservation of vital organs for later transplantation. Theologians, together with others, must therefore insist upon an open and thorough consideration of the following major options as viable options for the management of terminally ill patients or patients whose brain has suffered massive destruction to the extent of being irremediably nonfunctioning:

1. withdrawal of artificial and/or mechanical life-support systems (i.e., noninterference with death);

2. administration of pain-relieving drugs which will have the effect, among other effects, of accelerating the death process (i.e., hastening of death);

3. administration of death-inducing or life-terminating agents (i.e., deliberate action calculated to cause death).

There appears to be, among all the alternative opinions we have examined—medical, legal, and theological—a growing consensus that the terminally ill or irremediably injured patient should not have his death unreasonably or contemptibly prolonged. Where there is conflict, it has largely to do with the means whereby death is assisted; and it is for this reason that "indirect" or "passive" euthanasia is the form which presently enjoys widest

[55] Cf. Henry K. Beecher, et al., "A Definition of Irreversible Coma," Report of the Ad Hoc Committee at Harvard Medical School to Examine the Definition of Brain Death, Journal of the American Medical Association (1968), 205:337-40. The report states that (1) unreceptivity and unresponsitivity, (2) no movements or breathing, and (3) no reflexes are the characteristic signs of a permanently nonfunctioning brain, and that a flat or isoelectric EEG is confirmatory of the diagnosis. As a precautionary measure, the report advises that all these tests should be repeated at least 24 hours later, that if there is then no change in the data, and that if two further conditions (hypothermia and evidence of drug intoxication) are excluded, the patient may then be reasonably regarded as hopelessly and irreversibly damaged, and all those involved in major decisions affecting him so informed. Thereafter death is declared and supportive measures withdrawn.

[56] Supra, Chap. III, p. 108.

professional and public acceptance. It is, I think, self-evident that the values at stake in these options need considerably more extensive and detailed examination than they have thus far received. Meanwhile, however, employing the personal and interpersonal perspective from which we have viewed these matters, I think it arguable that options 1 and 2 are now morally licit procedures in the management of terminal or brain-destroyed patients, but that option 3 is not needed if we properly understand and apply the dispensability (i.e., the nonmandatoriness) of both extraordinary means and ordinary means which are not remedies. The line between options 2 and 3 is a fine one, I know; but it is reinforced by the awareness that medical science and technology have developed many possibilities for which we have not yet developed the ethical wisdom and moral stamina necessary for exercising humanely responsible control.

Index